MENTAL ILLNESS AND SOCIAL POLICY

THE AMERICAN EXPERIENCE

MENTAL ILLNESS AND SOCIAL POLICY

THE AMERICAN EXPERIENCE

TWENTIETH CENTURY PSYCHIATRY

Its Contribution to Man's Knowledge of Himself

William A[lanson] White

ARNO PRESS
A NEW YORK TIMES COMPANY
New York • 1973

Reprint Edition 1973 by Arno Press Inc.

Reprinted from a copy in
  The University of Illinois Library

MENTAL ILLNESS AND SOCIAL POLICY:
  The American Experience
ISBN for complete set: 0-405-05190-5
See last pages of this volume for titles.

Manufactured in the United States of America

————◆————

Library of Congress Cataloging in Publication Data

White, William Alanson, 1870-1937.
    Twentieth century psychiatry.

    (Mental illness and social policy: the American
experience)
    Reprint of the 1936 ed. published by Norton,
New York, in series: Thomas W. Salmon memorial
lectures, New York Academy of Medicine.
    Bibliography: p.
    1. Psychiatry. I. Title. II. Series.
III. Series: New York Academy of Medicine. Thomas
William Salmon memorial lectures.   [DNLM: WM100
W589t 1936F]
RC454.W49 1973   616.8'9   73-2428
ISBN 0-405-05236-7

TWENTIETH CENTURY PSYCHIATRY

Its Contribution to Man's Knowledge of Himself

44138

THOMAS W. SALMON MEMORIAL
LECTURES

DESTINY AND DISEASE IN
MENTAL DISORDERS
By Dr. C. Macfie Campbell

TWENTIETH CENTURY
PSYCHIATRY:
Its Contribution to Man's Knowledge
of Himself
By Dr. Wm. A. White

In Preparation

PSYCHOBIOLOGY
By Dr. Adolf Meyer

TWENTIETH CENTURY PSYCHIATRY

Its Contribution to Man's Knowledge of Himself

By WILLIAM A. WHITE

M.D., A.M., SC.D.

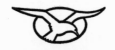

W. W. NORTON & COMPANY, INC.

Publishers, New York

PRINTED IN THE UNITED STATES OF AMERICA FOR THE
PUBLISHERS BY THE VAN REES PRESS

CONTENTS

PREFACE

I n presenting these lectures in book form I am again reminded of my difficulties in their preparation for delivery last year at The New York Academy of Medicine to a general audience. I of course could not know what the exact make-up of my audience would be but I naturally supposed—and as it turned out I think I was correct in this supposition—that it would be made up of some psychiatrists, some social workers, and a group of generally interested persons, some of whom might be laymen, some perhaps lawyers, some medical students, and perhaps others of various interests. It therefore became a problem as to just how the subject matter of psychiatry should be presented. It might have been made so highly technical that only a very small minority of the audience could have understood it, or it might have been

7

Preface

over-simplified to the point of being uninteresting and uninformative to those with technical qualifications and backgrounds of education and experience who were functioning in the psychiatric field in some capacity. Feeling as I did that the opportunity afforded me in giving these lectures was one which I wanted to utilize to the full in expressing my thoughts upon the various aspects of psychiatry as recently developed, I naturally was torn between the two extremes of a technical and a popular presentation of the subject. If, therefore, in an attempt to compose these differences and to get the best result from a compromise position between the two extremes I have at places been over-technical for the uninitiated and in other places over-simple for the initiated, I beg the reader, as I would in retrospect beg my audiences, to consider the difficulties under which I labored and out of such consideration to be lenient in their criticisms in this particular.

Washington, D. C.   W.A.W.

INTRODUCTION

IN THESE PAGES it shall be my object, first, to deal with psychiatry as a medical specialty; second, to discuss the social significance of psychiatry; and, third, to take up the general implications of psychiatric thought. In doing this I feel that I should indicate beforehand and at once the way in which I shall approach this task. In the first place, I shall not attempt to set forth the accomplishments of psychiatry either in chronological order or as being the individual contributions of particular personalities. My interests are somewhat other than these. They are functional in nature, and I shall present the subject from this point of view. Dates are elusive things. Pinel's liberation of the "insane" in 1792 and 1793 is an outstanding historical fact, more particularly, however, because of its dramatic setting,

9

for his act at that time by no means accomplished in other institutions and in other parts of the world the results that he obtained in the Paris hospitals. In fact over a century after this illustrious psychiatrist had, as it were, blazed the trail, Dr. Salmon reported conditions in one of the States of the Union which were as atrocious from the humanitarian point of view, and the result of as profound ignorance, as anything that Pinel uncovered in Paris. On the other hand, while it may be said of psychiatry, as of any other scientific discipline, that its historical progress is not only punctuated by dramatic events like that just mentioned but is dependent upon outstanding personalities, nevertheless, just as events only seem to be confined to specific periods of time, so progress as it is exemplified by personality similarly only seems to be adequately represented in this particular; for every great man not only stands upon the shoulders of his predecessors, but that which he is able to accomplish, either because of his peculiar qualifications or his fortunate circumstances, has already been prepared for him by preceding events. And so the really important thing so far as the subject matter of scientific progress itself is concerned is, in my mind, as I have already indicated, the story in its functional outlines.

In order that we may have some idea of psychiatry as a medical specialty of today it is desirable to know

Introduction

something of how this present-day psychiatry has arrived; in other words, what has been its history? A detailed history of psychiatry is of course out of the question as a matter of presentation in these lectures. Even a brief history is impossible. I merely call attention to what I believe to be a fact: that although an historical treatise on this subject would take us back to the earliest records, nevertheless all of the important things in psychiatry as we know it today have either happened or culminated during the past half century. Previous to that the movement of maximum significance was in the direction of the humanitarian care of the "insane"; since then the movement of maximum significance has been in the direction of scientific advancement of psychiatric knowledge. These two movements are not separated by a sharp line of demarcation. Care of the institutionalized cases of mental disease is still in a primitive state of development in many places in the world, whereas the scientific attitude toward mental disorder is still unknown in many aspects of our highest civilization; so that we may be prepared for finding all historical levels represented at any given time or place.

In the latter years of the nineteenth century the state of psychiatry, as I found it when I entered this field, is, I presume, hardly conceivable by the young man of today who starts upon the study of this specialty. The only mental diseases about which anything at all was known were those afflicting persons who were committed to public institutions, and here the knowledge for the most part was very primitive. It is true, of course, that at this time there were outstanding personalities here and in Europe that were far in advance of the group generally. This is always so, but it is not until the group catches up that their ideas really become of any considerable significance. And so at a time when the mind was, if anything, a greater mystery than it is today, when the study of psychology as a science had hardly begun and when it was still allied with the study of morals and of philosophy, when the parallelistic theory for the explanation of the relation between psychological and somatic events still ruled our thinking, we were in a state not of progress, but one might say of stagnation, that it is well to contemplate whenever we feel discouraged because of the slowness of our progress. I often state, and I verily believe, that no department of medicine has advanced with the rapidity of psychiatry. Forty-three years ago, when I entered the New York State service, as a medical specialty psychiatry hardly existed, and the average hospital psychiatrist was little if any removed in his understanding of mental cases from the ward attendant, and far less informed than the present-day psychiatric social worker, although this latter comparison I realize is hardly a fair one to the psychiatrist. Such scientific efforts as were made consisted of a combination of clinical work at the purely descriptive level with a pathology that was entirely of the dead-house variety. Taking this combination in connection with a mystical idea of mind which considered it as something inexplicable, running along parallel to the manifestations of the body but being uninfluenced by them and uninfluencing them in turn, one can perhaps get some faint idea of the terrific handicaps with which the student in this field had to contend in those days. And when it came to matters of therapy, here the limitations were just as great. All therapy in those days was a therapy of negation. Restraint of one form or another was the order of the day; and even if the doctrine of non-restraint was under discussion, as it was in these early days, still only the elect had the remotest idea of what this doctrine of non-restraint involved. If patients did anything that it was presumed they ought not to do, the idea was to interfere with that doing and to prevent it if possible. Physical restraint of all kinds and descriptions was in vogue for violent conduct. This form of restraint was to a considerable extent in the course of these years substituted by chemical restraint, which was just as bad because the drugs that were used were delirium-producing drugs. Every effort of this sort that was made, restraint by physical, chemical or in other ways, direct or indirect, in the last analysis produced the very results which it aimed at avoiding. The patient physically restrained became so resentful of his environment, physical and personal alike, that he was ready for destructive and assaultive conduct at any time at a moment's notice or at the slightest suggestion. The patient chemically restrained was in a constant state of confusion and semi-delirium, during which he became a much more difficult problem to care for than he would have been otherwise. And so our institutions, which you must remember were the only places where mental disorder was really seen at all, became collections, on the one hand, of violent and destructive and instinctually unrelated individuals, and, on the other hand, a small group of persons who had come through with considerable success and who were trusted and efficient members of the hospital family—patients who had parole, patients who did work on the farm or were able consistently to employ themselves in other capacities. This was the material upon which modern psychiatry had to found. These were the beginnings out of which we have reached our present estate. These days contained the plan from which we have developed our present structure and undoubtedly they have contributed elements to that structure, some of which, at least, we are not at all clearly conscious of.

In order that we may further realize the situation as it then existed I will take a chapter from the study of the feebleminded and apply it to the institutionalized "insane." It will be recalled that our opinions about the feebleminded have changed very materially during the present century. We used to think that feebleminded individuals were fundamentally and essentially dangerous, that they formed a group of society from which the criminals were largely recruited, that they easily became murderers, sex offenders, and perpetrators of other heinous offenses; and we got this idea very naturally because the only feebleminded people we saw were the occasional offenders of this kind who came into the public eye as a result of the commission of such deeds. When, however, we came to study the feebleminded problem in a scientific way and had tools by which we could measure, however roughly, the level of mental development of the individual, we learned that these feebleminded people that we had heretofore known were really exceptional and that our concept of feeblemindedness had been based solely upon this exceptional few. It is an exactly analogous situation in which we found ourselves with reference to the mentally ill at the end of the nineteenth century. The only mentally ill people we recognized were those who had been committed to public institutions, generally as a result of conduct which was grossly pathological, and so naturally our concepts of what constituted mental disease were formed accordingly.

It is perhaps not too much to say, when we consider the situation as I have described it, that the mentally ill were treated very much like animals. I do not say this critically, nor do I mean that they were treated with intentional cruelty. I mean by this that we had no more conception in those days of how to deal with a given symptom such as violence than we had how to deal with such a symptom in an animal. Psychopathology as we think of it today was practically non-existent and psychology gave us not the slightest assistance. We were forced, therefore, to draw upon our own personal experience and that invariably resulted in this frustration method of treatment because that is naturally the only thing that could possibly issue from such a restricted viewpoint as we necessarily had. Violence must be restrained. Bad habits must be discouraged by all manner of restrictive means. Everything must be done to insure against crimes, injuries and the like, with the result that nothing succeeded and the whole situation was aggravated inconceivably. Out of this welter of ignorance, fear and superstition, which combined in various proportions and in various ways in different individuals to produce these results, something had to eventuate, because matters had reached their limit in the direction of the creation of impossible conditions. The hospital was under suspicion from all quarters. Public criticism was addressed against it. Patients and their relatives feared it and refused, if possible, to avail themselves of its good offices. Perhaps the most significant thing that happened at this time, and which was a movement which even yet I do not believe has been adequately appreciated, was the "no restraint" movement. The history of this movement is well known. I will not dwell upon it. I merely wish to make the following brief comment upon it: that as soon as the principle of no restraint came to be applied this is what happened—a violent patient could not be restrained and for the first time those who were responsible for his care had to use their brains for this purpose. Necessarily when camisoles, strong sheets, handcuffs and the like were removed something had to take their place, and that something was intelligence. I doubt that this aspect of the no restraint movement has ever been adequately appreciated, but it is to my mind the significant nub of the whole situation.

From the time that this principle was accepted it necessarily resulted in a continuing improvement in the care of the institutionalized patient and a continuing improvement in the intelligence with which this care was administered by the personnel of the hospital. It is perhaps doubtful if we would have reached as far as we have today in our understanding of our mentally ill patients if this particular reform in their care had not been many years in developing by the time we began the investigation of mental disease along what we now call scientific lines.

In these early days, by which I refer to the latter part of the nineteenth century, one of the subjects that occupied the minds of the young institution psychiatrists—and there were no others—was the subject of the classification of mental diseases. As I look back upon these times I feel that this interest in classification had a deeper significance than I appreciated at the time. It was evidence of a deep-seated dissatisfaction with the existing knowledge of mental disorders and the result of a consequent feeling of discontent and unrest.[1] One of the first questions that would be asked a visiting psychiatrist from another institution would be, What classification do you use? When it is remembered that for the most part classifications were exceedingly simple and brief with very few subdivisions, the significance of this attitude will be apparent. I mention this matter of classification as it was thought of in those days because I believe that the attitude of the psychiatrists, their discontent with existing conditions, was one of reaching out toward what appeared to them the direction in which satisfactions might come; and it was because of this that when the Kraepelinian contribution, particularly as set forth in the sixth edition of Kraepelin's *Lehrbuch* (1899), came to the attention of the psychiatrists, as it did very shortly afterward and in the first few years of the

---

[1] Möbius, P. J.: *Die Hoffnungslosigkeit aller Psychologie*. Halle. C. Marhold. 1907. Discussed by Adolf Meyer in the *Psychological Bulletin*, Vol. 4, No. 6, June 15, 1907.

succeeding century through English translations, they seized upon it as presenting a new classification and were especially keen about the two great groups of dementia precox and the manic-depressive psychoses. Following upon this outstanding contribution to clinical psychiatry the whole subject of classification, in this country at least, largely lost interest, and today one hears very little of it. I do not need to labor the point here that classifications and definitions are merely tools for handling the material included therein, and that as information changes so must classifications and definitions. The point I would make, however, is that so long as the information and general state of knowledge of psychiatry were hopelessly unsatisfactory, and for reasons which I have indicated, the matter of classification in point of interest held the center of the stage. Now, however, with this vitalizing contribution of Kraepelin the whole subject of clinical psychiatry was vivified and transformed into a field of great interest, and correspondingly we hear very little about the subject of classification. The needs have been satisfied—not, to be sure, by new classifications. The tendency in that direction was a false trail and psychiatry is now embarked upon a new era and from this time forth continues to be surpassingly interesting and capable of capturing the imagination of the scientific mind.

Other events of surpassing importance to the

future of psychiatry were happening in these same years—the latter part of the nineteenth century and the first years of the present century. Kraepelin's contribution, as I have already mentioned, had a tremendous effect throughout the psychiatric world. As we will come to see later, however, Kraepelin fell far short of what we conceive today to be an adequate grasp of the possibilities, although this is by no means intended in any way to detract from the magnificent dimensions of his contribution. This was fundamental and continues to be fundamental. Without it it is difficult to see just how we would have attained our present stature. But his psychiatry remained at the descriptive level. Albeit he himself reached the highest point of development in this field of clinical description, he also appreciated the necessity of attacking the problem of mental disease from many directions instead of from a single direction; and he accumulated about him, especially after he left Heidelberg and went to Munich, a group of enthusiastic workers along these different lines. Where he fell short, after all, was in his basic concept that the mystery of the psychoses was to be unraveled by a study of their course and outcome. While this was an immense advance upon the previous cross-section method of clinical study, it was still hamstrung by the concept of disease then prevalent. Dementia precox, manic-depressive psychoses and paranoia were disease entities, and therefore the biological method of study, as he took it to be, could be applied to them properly. He failed to realize, as we do so thoroughly today, that the longitudinal section should include the entire life of the individual, of which the disease is an expression, and that even beyond that it should include the history of the phylum of which he is a part. There was no scale of values in this psychiatry from the point of view that we consider values today.

Following the projection of the Kraepelinian ideas psychiatry had a period of a number of years of great productivity. Interest was maintained at a high pitch and investigators all over the world began to create a voluminous literature following Kraepelin's lead. Extensive monographs appeared covering the main nosological entities, and correlations were sought with the stimulating and advancing work that was being done in pathology. Kraepelin himself also contributed a number of important studies of a psychological character, worthy predecessors of the work now being done along numerous lines in testing, which is at present in full blast. The little group at Munich dominated the psychiatric world, and No. 7 Nussbaumstrasse became the Mecca for psychiatrists the world over.

About this time, that is during the early years of the present century, there appeared those very wonderful studies of the feebleminded by Doctors Binet and Simon, and their development of their measuring scale for intelligence. Up to the time of the fabrication of this very important tool for measuring intelligence there had been no way of identifying the feebleminded in the community, and as a result they were not identified, and so the only knowledge existing regarding them was of the very malignant institution types. Now the whole subject of feeblemindedness was born anew. Feebleminded children were discovered in the school systems particularly, and the enormous importance of the problem of feeblemindedness began to be appreciated.

The development of a measuring rod for intelligence which made possible the discovery of the feebleminded in the community was followed rapidly by an appreciation of the social significance of this group, which was soon discovered to be very large—comparable in size to the group of the so-called insane. It was soon found that many of the social inadequacies of individuals were traceable to defects of intelligence. In fact social maladjustment of all sorts began to be attributed to this defect, and so the problems of crime, of poverty, of prostitution, were in turn investigated from this point of view, with the result that under the first flush of these new discoveries almost every conceivable social disability was attributed to intelligence defect. This somewhat exaggerated attitude and relatively simplistic explanation of all the troubles of the world might of course be expected under the circumstances. The discovery of new facts is very apt to be followed by their over-valuation. Nevertheless it was in work of this sort that perhaps the most significant contribution that this country has made to the whole problem of mental disorder and defect came into being, namely, the contribution which has been made to the social significance of these states and to the methods of dealing with them along social lines. In other words, as Dr. Salmon himself used to emphasize in the latter years of his life, it was to the social significance of mental disease that this country made its great contribution.

If the reader will follow these three lectures through to the end he will, I hope, discover gradually unfolding to his vision not only a concept of psychiatry in its more limited sense as a medical specialty but in that broader sense which relates it to all the other departments of thought and experience; and thus of necessity he will also discover that there is at the foundation of this presentation a philosophy in accordance with which its details are developed and differentiated. This philosophy, the author hopes, will be found to be helpful not only in the restricted area of the practice of psychiatry but in the whole field of medicine, not to say the still broader field of human relations. It is with this hope that these lectures have been delivered and now appear in book form.

I

PSYCHIATRY

AS A MEDICAL

SPECIALTY

BEFORE PLUNGING INTO the subject of psychiatry, which I shall present in the pages of this book, I cannot refrain from what seems to me a very illuminating reference to Dr. Thomas W. Salmon, to whom I owe, through the medium of the memorial established in his name, the opportunity of making this presentation. The incident which I have in mind took place, I should say, about twenty years ago on the occasion of a public meeting—I believe it was one of the annual luncheons of the National Committee for Mental Hygiene held for the purpose of giving opportunity for a more or less public discussion of the general subject of mental health and the prevention of mental disease. Dr. Salmon was there and of course it came his turn to speak. I can see him now, in my mind's eye, as he stands there addressing the audience. His visual image possesses all of the characteristics which belonged to him in life, particularly that very individual smile of his with which he accompanied the presentation of his thesis, and his very characteristic, slow-spoken and convincing manner of utterance. I can hear him saying, as if it were yesterday, that "Psychiatry is the Cinderella of Medicine"; and I am wondering, if he were alive to-day, what he would say as to its present status, for far from being a Cinderella, in the minds of a great many people, particularly those who are in need of its services, it is now, in their wishful thinking, the Fairy Godmother, who, by a wave of her wand and perhaps the pronouncement of a few magic words, can work the miracles which they desire.

I can well remember when I entered the New York State service, the State Care Act was just coming into force. This act provided that the state take over the care of the so-called insane, and, therefore, by implication, it took them from the poor-houses and the jails into the great state hospitals. These hospitals, which, by the way, had only recently acquired that name and had previously been known as asylums, therefore became the repositories of the mentally ill of the entire state. When I took service in one of them I found myself in an entirely new sort of world. I had recently completed an interneship in a general hospital and had been accustomed to the routine of medical, surgical, obstetrical

26

and children's wards, the operating room, the dispensary, the ambulance service, and here I found none of these. The wards were provided with no special equipment for the practice of medicine and each one of us had to function much like the reputed country doctor and attend to whatever happened to any one of his many, usually several hundred, patients. Our standard equipment consisted of a percussion hammer, a stethoscope and a thermometer, and with these, plus a little pocket case that my preceptor had given me, I undertook the practice of medicine and psychiatry. Even those of us who were sufficiently industrious to try to find some assistance from the fields of cerebral anatomy and physiology and from psychology sought in those directions in vain. Few of our patients had any demonstrable lesions of the nervous system and psychology seemed to know nothing of our problems. In striking contrast to our poverty, not only of equipment but of ideas, of those days, I pick up a copy of Kretschmer's *Medical Psychology* that recently came to my desk, and read in the Translator's Introduction that: "It is a compendium of empirical facts and observations derived from anatomy, physiology, neurology, biochemistry, epistemology, psychiatry, psychoanalysis (and allied schools), folk-psychology, biology, anthropology, aesthetics, and many other sources, systematically arranged in such a way as to throw a great deal of light on the problems of human thought, feeling, and

27

conduct in health and disease." This surely represents a stupendous change that has come about in
what seems a remarkably short period of time, so
short in fact as to represent an advance in this field
that is little short of miraculous and which, I am
sure you will agree with me, compares very favorably
with the advance in other departments of medicine.

Naturally I cannot cover all aspects of such a
large subject as the medical specialty of psychiatry.
It would be foolish even to attempt to do so. I shall
undertake only to discuss, somewhat disconnectedly
I fear, certain of its aspects which appear to be especially significant for one reason or another.

At the turn of the century two great movements
arose, both of which were destined to become of
profound significance in the development of psychiatry and both of which remain of great significance
for the future. These two movements were the psychoanalytic movement and the mental hygiene movement. I mention them together because it would seem
that what has happened in the field of psychiatry
could hardly be understood by considering either one
alone. While in many respects they have little in
common, nevertheless they supplement each other
in very fundamental ways. I will take up the psychoanalytic movement first, asking you to realize that
no linear description of the progress of psychiatry
is possible, that many things are happening con-
temporaneously along different lines of progress,

and that in a lecture of this sort it is impossible to reproduce the complexity of the pattern as it proceeds to unfold.

The psychoanalytic movement made its appearance in the early years of the century and was represented in this country by a very small group of men, who organized the first society in 1911 (New York Psychoanalytic Society). They were very fortunate from the beginning to enlist the support of Dr. James J. Putnam and Professor G. Stanley Hall. Mature men with the wisdom of experience and with many years of outstanding accomplishments to their credit, their connection with the movement served to soften a great deal of the bitter antagonism which developed against it from the very earliest days, particularly, as you well know, because of its emphasis upon sex. However, like all new movements, it was enthusiastically sponsored, although not always wisely, by the younger members, who frequently unnecessarily gave openings for attacks and who were not always judicious. The movement in its beginning suffered from these disabilities and from a certain rawness which is apt to be found where youth and enthusiasm are mixed. I am reminded of what Whitehead says: "It is a well-founded historical generalization, that the last thing to be discovered in any science is what the science is really about. Men go on groping for centuries, guided merely by a dim instinct and a puzzled curiosity, till at last 'some great truth is loosened.' " [1] And so in these early days there was a great deal of groping and puzzled curiosity, which was compensated for by youth and enthusiasm and which was based upon an intuitive feeling of certainty that we were on the right track.

As I look back upon those days I feel that Professor Freud was quite right in his sizing up of the American situation when he said, in substance, that he felt more apprehensive for psychoanalysis in this country than elsewhere because it was received with open arms, and (here is the point) too uncritically. It is not good for ideas to be accepted without criticism. Criticism represents the difficulties that have to be overcome, and new movements like psychoanalysis need all the criticism they can get because they need the strength that comes only from surmounting obstacles. In fact I have heard it said by one of the most eminent of our American analysts that now that analysis was being progressively better and better received by the scientific world and had won its fight against the criticism that it was involved entirely and completely in the elaboration of the sex instinct in its studies, that the next great obstacle it would encounter, a greater one than it had met heretofore, would be the real, true test of its strength, when people found out what analysis really

[1] Whitehead, A. N.: *An Introduction to Mathematics.* New York. Henry Holt & Co. 1911.

meant, what it really involved and what its true significance was. I have had this possibility impressed upon me recently when I received a letter from the Middle West asking me to find a son who had disappeared from his family and intimating that my science—whatever it was in their minds, I am not sure—might enable me to do it. It must be remembered that the public, at least the afflicted portion of it who need help, would like to have that help come in the form of magic. They would wish to go to the doctor's office, have him write a mysterious prescription in an unknown tongue, in which they were directed to take a certain amount at certain times in the day and then have everything rapidly become perfectly all right, have all their troubles disappear without having themselves to have done anything whatever about it. We cannot get anything in this world without paying for it in one way or another; and I think there will be as much resentment against paying the price for mental health as there obviously is for paying the price for physical health, but when the time comes the price will have to be paid nevertheless. I am glad at this point to be able to state that the American Psychiatric Association has constituted a Section on Psychoanalysis. This I believe to be a step in the right direction, for it will require the psychoanalytic communications of this section to be presented in open forum, where they will receive the just and proper criticism of the psychiatric group and fall into their proper place at least as instruments of therapeutic procedure in relation to the general body of psychiatry.

Much has happened, however, since those early days. The number of workers in this field has steadily increased, and, particularly, the preparation with which the workers have entered the field has been constantly improved, so that the workers throughout the world are now a goodly number of well trained individuals who are contributing in ever increasing amounts to the literature. As you know, however, this work has not directly as yet been of any great service in the field of the therapy of the malignant psychoses. The schizophrenias and the manic-depressives still present practically unsolvable problems for the psychoanalytic technique. This, however, does not mean that nothing has been gained by psychiatry from this field; quite the contrary is the case. For the first time, really, in the history of psychiatry, meanings and values were introduced into the understanding of the psychoses. Description naturally has its place, but dynamic concepts based upon the significance of psychological symptoms have crowded mere description and classification almost off the map. And even if, roughly speaking, the institutional psychiatrist is no more able to cure his patients than he was twenty-five years ago, he approaches them now with interest and with some considerable measure of understanding; and this, after all, is the first

A Medical Specialty

and most important step for the solving of these enormously important social problems. I sometimes think that if a problem can be formulated that is the most important step that can be taken, because after the problem is formulated, when it is known what the problem is, where it is, something of its boundaries, its limitations, its difficulties and their nature, then it can be left to the natural curiosity and creative efforts of man to produce sooner or later a solution. And so psychiatry has been greatly blessed by the psychoanalytic movement in these ways. Its problems have been more clearly defined, they are more definitely understood, their meanings and values have become significant, and the patient in each instance is receiving more intelligent consideration and in the end I have no doubt that the net result will be a definite gain in therapeutic results.

Even so much as has already been attained, however, has been attained under the greatest difficulties and in opposition to the most virulent criticisms. "Mankind has a poor ear for new music." [2] The psychiatrists of the future, like those of the past, must, however, continue to guard the interests of their patients as their primary concern and so approach all claims with an open mind, determined to discard all considerations of a personal or prejudicial nature and to garner from all the material presented

[2] Nietzsche.

all that can be put to good use for the purposes at hand.

I am not going into all these matters except in so far as they seem to be pertinent to my purposes. One of the criticisms which is addressed against analysis and that body of knowledge which has grown up around it as a nucleus, is that it is not scientific because it cannot formulate its results quantitatively. It is believed by some that nothing is worth while that cannot be stated in a mathematical formula. I merely pause long enough to mention this criticism because it seems to have captured the imagination of a certain important group, and I am thinking of the universities. As Miss Goodenough very aptly says:[3] "No science would progress far if it refused to use imperfect tools when no others were available."[4] However, I will not attempt to criticize mathematicians because I know too little about mathematics. And that is just the point. They should not criticize us because they know nothing about our problems either. The methodology of psychiatry, and particularly the technique of psychoanalysis, was produced for therapeutic purposes. Now the fact happens to be that patients who are subjected to this

[3] *Developmental Psychology*. Pub. by D. Appleton & Co., 1934.

[4] It would be as sensible to have criticized the mathematicians for not employing the symbols of the calculus before the days of Newton and Leibnitz.

A Medical Specialty

procedure do get well. The only quarrel can be over the explanation of the process of getting well, or the correctness of the formulations upon which it is based. And here again I will quote Whitehead, who with reference to this whole question, the possibility of a correct solution coming out of wrong premises, says: "It is this possibility of being right, albeit with entirely wrong explanations as to what is being done, that so often makes external criticism—that is so far as it is meant to stop the pursuit of a method—singularly barren and futile in the progress of science." [5]

Back of all this, however, there is a real, substantial and adequate reason for criticism of the constructive sort. The thing that befuddles the physicist as he approaches these problems with his entirely different point of view and different training is their intangibility and lack of objectivity; and if his criticism means that we should attempt to make our work more specific, concrete if you will, and objective, then that is all right, the point is well taken, and as a matter of fact our methods and techniques are moving in this direction.

Meanwhile it would be well if the most severe critic of psychoanalysis were to be the psychoanalyst himself; and with that rare, unprejudiced, critical ability which is a part of the well trained, well balanced scientific mind he should go forward with his researches unhampered by any other motive than

[5] *Loc. cit.*

the search for truth, realizing that this rather gratuitous and unmerited criticism that nothing is of any value unless it can be measured, like many other things is of perhaps little account. Nothing gets to be measurable until it passes through many intermediate stages of development on the way, and the quicker we get to work at these intermediate stages the sooner the goal, if goal it be, will be reached.

It would be a consummation devoutly to be wished if the universities would recognize research in this field by taking on workers and freeing them from the necessity of anything but a life of research. In this way progress could be stimulated in a very wholesome, worth while way with valuable results.

The outstanding goal of our efforts, as I see them today and as they are represented by the psychoanalytic school, is to build up slowly and painstakingly an anatomy and a physiology of the psyche comparable in exactness of its outlines and complexity of its structures to the anatomy and physiology of the body. If our thinking is moving along in the right direction we must believe that bodily and mental states are not either separate or different from one another but are only two aspects of the organism-as-a-whole, from either one of which we may view its activities. If this is so, as I have reiterated so many times, then the history of the psyche reaches as far into the past as that of the soma, and for each state of one there is a corresponding repercussion in the other.[6] This means that our knowledge of psychological affairs will be as intricately involved as our knowledge of bodily affairs; and the principal significance of this statement is to point to the fact that as regards the affairs of the psyche we have only begun to gain that knowledge. The surface has

[6] One of the great difficulties in expressing the new point of view here advocated is that it has to be expressed in the language which was evolved for the purposes of expressing the point of view which is now being discarded. To try to express that body and mind are merely different aspects of the organism and not different things is difficult in a language in which "body" and "mind" are both substantives and where the theory is that a noun is a thing. No doubt, however, new terms will arise or new meanings will gradually take the place of the old meanings so that this difficulty will gradually disappear, but in any case language, as indicated in this instance, becomes a real obstacle to the expression of new concepts. The best, probably, that can be done at present is to have a recognition and understanding of this difficulty.

Commenting upon this disability of language for describing what occurs within the atom, Heisenberg says: "It is not surprising that our language should be incapable of describing the processes occurring within the atoms, for, as has been remarked, it was invented to describe the experiences of daily life, and these consist only of processes involving exceedingly large numbers of atoms. Furthermore, it is very difficult to modify our language so that it will be able to describe these atomic processes, for words can only describe things of which we can form mental pictures, and this ability, too, is a result of daily experience."

37

only been scratched. Some, probably, of the fundamental directions and tendencies have been outlined, but as to the great mass of detailed superstructure, its understanding is a thing mostly for the future. I do not believe that after careful consideration, for example, of Abraham's stages in libido development —important as they have been, enlightening as they are, developed as they were for psychotherapeutic purposes on the basis of psychopathological types of reaction—that anyone can say that they make even a pretense at completeness. They are a beginning statement which indicates only possibilities—possibilities which in their unfolding may change the face of things as we see them now very, very largely.

To give some idea of the importance and significance of the issues, even so far as the principles have been at present uncovered, I refer to a recent communication of Money Kyrle [7] wherein he questions whether aggression is an independent impulse of the nature of an instinct, as Freud believes, and states that "although the most offensive of Freud's theories have usually been found to be correct" he still finds himself unconvinced with regard to this particular one. I shall not undertake a discussion of this question but merely call it to your attention. The whole matter of the aggressive instinct as set forth by Freud, and particularly the death instinct, has

[7] Kyrle, R. Money: "A Psychologist's Utopia." *Psyche.* April 1931.

been a very valuable contribution and has helped greatly to elucidate our thinking with respect to certain types of thinking and behavior. Nevertheless, if aggression is the ingrained, instinctive sort of thing that Freud thinks it is, he is entirely warranted in his depressed and somewhat pessimistic attitude toward the future. If, on the other hand, it is, as Money Kyrle thinks, a reaction to frustration, then surely there is much to be hoped for, because frustrating forces can be attacked. Frustrations, academically at least, are capable of being cured if the conditions which produce them can be done away with. Here is a fundamental, significant and important issue. In these changing and disturbing times it is important that we should occasionally take stock of all the advantages that modern science has placed at our disposal and ask whether we may not be living in a fool's paradise when we assume without question that everything that happens is in the direction of progress, that we are moving as a whole towards levels of higher civilization, that man is evolving in all his parts toward better things. We know perfectly well from the history of organic life as exhibited in other forms than man that an uninterrupted progressive development is not by any means always the rule, and we need therefore to ask ourselves what we may have lost in this process of civilization. But these are questions that are easier asked than answered and the discussion of which alone would be sufficient, even in the most abbreviated form, to occupy this whole lecture.

In any consideration of the psychoanalytic movement it should always be borne in mind that the criticisms which have been aimed at it, or at least those criticisms which were emotionally conditioned and most severe and were especially directed against its so-called pan-sexual tendencies, were criticisms that were aimed at the content of what was disclosed by the psychoanalytic method and not at the process or the mechanism or the form, as you will, of the neurosis or psychosis as the case might be. This criticism of the highly individualistic content that was disclosed can be seen, I think easily, to be of much less significance than would a like severity of criticism of the psychological processes. This conclusion, I believe, necessarily follows because, after all, content is largely exquisitely personal, depending upon the past experiences of a particular individual; and the deeper the analysis goes and the less personal the content comes to be, the more important becomes the process or the mechanisms. In other words, the material becomes more impersonal as it approaches those features which are common to everybody and which likewise become more and more nearly of an organic nature. The deeper the analysis goes the less significance has the individual material and the greater significance the mechanisms, and therefore, in conformity with my own predilections, the more nearly the whole situation can be expressed in terms of energy exchange.

One of the best examples of the usefulness of the energy concept is very well illustrated in a recent article by Dr. Karin Stephen.[8] She discusses more particularly those feelings, with which we are all familiar and which are expressed delusionally, of being the host more generally of malignant influences—sometimes beneficent but usually not—influences that are felt to be harming the patient or influences, on the other hand, which the patient feels are emanating from him and are destructive to those about. These influences are personified oftentimes as enemies, or they are considered in a more mystical way as being evil spirits, but their outstanding peculiarity is that they are definite forces which inhabit or invade the patient and have a specific and concrete existence of their own. There are two outstanding characteristics of the developmental stages in the infantile and child psyche which help us to understand these phenomena. In the first place, this period of the early months corresponds rather closely to the animistic period of culture, and the child like the savage in that stage has great difficulty in differentiating himself from the environment. What is "I" and what is "not I" is still a rather con-

[8] Stephen, Karin: "Introjection and Projection: Guilt and Rage." *Brit. Jr. of Medical Psychology,* Vol. XIV, Part IV, 1934.

fused conglomerate, and the differentiation is something which has to be learned by painful experience. Therefore distressing internal states cannot be determined, to begin with, as coming either from within or without. The other and in some respects more significant assistance to understanding this condition, especially in using the energy concept, is that these forces or spirits or influences, or whatever they may be called, which the patient feels inside of him, have their origin in visceral activities and emotional explosions, either or both, and which when they occur are felt by the child as being something uncontrollable, and because uncontrollable it takes a long period of experience before they can be identified as activities of the self. Consequently when these experiences are distressing they are easily, in this animistic period, identified as evil possessions, influences, or what not, and the contrary when they are pleasurable; and on the other hand, with the lack of definition as to their origin, it is as easy for them to be conceived as emanating from without as from within. And so this whole host of feelings and influences which are so familiar in our psychiatric experience receives for the first time anything approaching an adequate explanation by the mechanisms that psychoanalysis has uncovered. As Dr. Stephen says regarding this whole field of phenomena: "I know of no theory which even attempts an

A Medical Specialty

explanation other than the one offered by psycho-analysis."

You will see that this explanation fits in, with slight modifications of terminology, to the energy concept which I like so much.[9] In connection herewith I would call your attention to the work of the Chicago group under Alexander [10] who are investigating a certain group of diseases, particularly of the digestive system, which have always been considered organic but which evidence many reasons for believing that there are at least important psychogenic factors in the etiology. The formulations of the results which they have reached thus far are related to the three main functions of the gastro-intestinal tract which its subdivisions so definitely classify. These are the functions of taking the food in, of digestion and all that implies, and of excretion, or, as it might be put more briefly, the functions of ingestion, digestion and egestion. You will see that these last three terms indicate that they are special

[9] I am of course familiar with the theory that attributes to these forces when they are anthropomorphized their origin in the parental imagines, but it seems to me that this is peculiarly individual material and not as significant or fundamental as the underlying mechanism as explained above.

[10] Alexander, F., Bacon C., Levey, H., Levine M., Wilson, G. W.: "Symposium on the Influence of Psychologic Factors upon Gastro-Intestinal Disturbances." *Psychoanalytic Quarterly,* Vol. III, No. 4. October 1934.

instances of the handling of energy by the organism, which Dr. Jelliffe and I have insisted upon and have classified also in a similar way as the capture, transformation and delivery of energy. The substitution of energy for food is perfectly legitimate in these days of modern physics. Such general statements of the functions of the organism on the face of them might be supposed to be too general to be of value, but taken in connection with what appears to be necessary to an understanding of the organism, the division into general and special which appears from time to time with different names to designate these two features, such as particulate and diffuse, or localized and multipotential, it can be seen that we are dealing with a very similar concept in its various manifestations and that to understand the organism from the point of view of the processes of differentiation it is essential to have a background of this more general, or, as I often call it, protoplasmic concept of the material and forces out of which this differentiation emerges.

Another very important and significant feature of the whole psychoanalytic movement has been the disclosure of the fact that every illness has its psychological component, so that in a sense it will be seen that psychiatry is the one medical specialty which in its broadest conception can be seen to be the central point of all the other medical specialties; for it is only from the standpoint of the psychiatrist, or, perhaps better, from the psychological level, that the significance of disease of the various parts of the body can be understood. From this point of view we get an integrated concept of the organism and an understanding of its purposes which cannot be derived from any partial examination of the functions of a particular organ.

And I may add with regard to the psychoanalytic movement that if it were not for the contributions from this source psychiatry would be entirely without a clue to the meanings of many symptoms, and, while not without therapeutic resources, without very much hope as to the efficacy of these resources in many of the more serious and more malignant situations with which we have to deal. So much of our understanding of the symptomatology of mental disorder has come from psychoanalytic sources that I believe that in the future the main contribution psychoanalysis will make to psychiatry is in the uncovering of the meanings of symptoms, because it is through their understanding that any adequate treatment plan must be developed.

Perhaps the most important contribution to the understanding and meaning of psychological symptomatology will come as a result of the contribution that psychoanalysis is able to make by way of character analysis and its resulting significance for the further elaboration of the whole subject of typology. It is in this field of what has been called depth analysis that we may expect to be able to find some indications that will assist us in differentiating the part played in certain symptoms by heredity on the one hand or identification on the other. This I conceive to be a really important question. We see so many patients who have symptoms almost identical with those of a parent, for example, and yet the symptoms appear to be at least largely functional. The question is, Are these symptoms conditioned by hereditary factors or are they the result of the mechanism of identification? Or, perhaps, a third supposition, which is still more probable, Do they come about through an interplay of both of these factors?

Finally, it must be recognized regarding psychoanalysis that despite the apparent opinions of some of its advocates, it does not offer a methodology which at the present time should be thought of as replacing all others in the field of psychopathology. There are many approaches to the problems of the mind and each one has its contributions to make to their solution; and it is quite natural, and in fact inevitable, that each method should pursue its own course in accordance with its own rules, standards and ideals, and it is hardly necessary for me to say that we cannot expect all these different methods to harmonize at any particular time. We have to realize that the field of psychopathology is larger than any one of them and that in so doing we should remain tolerant to all points of view and particularly receptive to all contributions. At the present time I believe the psychoanalytic point of view can be said unequivocally to have made the most important contribution in this field, but, quite in harmony with scientific progress elsewhere, it has raised more questions than it has solved and tomorrow the emphasis may lie somewhere else. We must be prepared to follow the course of scientific unfoldment wherever it may lead. We need every tool, every method, every avenue of approach, every dexterity that we can devise, and therefore we should be as alert in recognizing facts in other regions of thought, facts uncovered by other methods, as some of us are now in defending the very specific procedures of psychoanalytic therapy. At any rate, any fair evaluation of psychoanalysis must consider it as a body of expanding, developing knowledge. One who has lived through in experience its relation to psychiatry can hardly fail to appreciate its invaluable contribution and be convinced of its future possibilities.

It is, of course, quite impossible to discuss in detail the problem of therapeutics as related to the psychoses, but at this point it seems to me to be worth while to call attention to the fact that psychoanalysis of course is by no means the only available form of therapy. For a long time, especially for the relatively minor psychological disturbances, particularly for hysteria, hypnosis in some of its variations held sway as being considered by some the method of choice; but hypnosis, despite the fact that it has certain definite qualifications for certain situations, is out of style, for unfortunately custom rules in this field as well as therapeutic experience. In mentioning hypnosis, however, I cannot let the subject pass without saying that the whole field that is covered by this term, which includes the entire field of the operation of suggestion, is one of very considerable significance and one which it seems to me lends itself peculiarly to research along the lines of the uncovering of the significance of certain phenomena. I will mention only two. Throughout the field of psychotherapy there are from time to time reported cases in which changes that have been wrought in the psychological mechanisms have been accompanied by changes in the somatic systems which at times have been little less than miraculous. Carefully regulated and controlled experiments in the field of hypnosis and suggestibility could be arranged in the laboratory, in my opinion, that would throw tremendously important light upon this whole subject, a subject which not only needs illumination in order to satisfy our natural curiosity regarding such things but which goes very deeply in connection with many important methods. There is probably no therapy, drug therapy or surgical therapy or any other kind, that has not its component of influence exercised at the psychological level. Every form of therapy is administered by a personality. We can never have too much information about the extent and the character of the mechanisms of these psychological influences. Then, too, there are many phenomena which at present we are unable to put in their proper category. There are many important and significant questions upon which experimental work in the field of hypnosis would, I think, throw important light. Another question of outstanding importance is that of the relation at the psychological level of the physician to his patient, with the understanding and acknowledgment of the fact, which rarely seems to be mentioned, that the experimenter or the physician in every such position is a part and parcel of the very problem which he is undertaking to solve. This, however, is only a special case of the broad principle that in all of man's efforts to explain and understand himself he cannot objectify the problems in accordance with the demands of the physical sciences. He is a part of what he is trying to explain: a fact that those same physical sciences will have to take more serious note of in the future. This fact makes all contributions in the field of psychotherapy peculiarly subject to artifacts and peculiarly difficult. In the field of hypnosis, where the whole situation is more or less under definite control and where experiments can be devised specifically to answer definite questions rather than having to wait for Nature to present an experiment to us in the way of illness, these matters might receive consideration that would advance our learning. I offer these suggestions because I feel that this entire field of study needs to be stimulated, and because it is not only out of fashion but temporarily, at least, and to some extent, certainly is not in good repute scientifically.

If psychoanalysis had never made but one contribution to our thinking it would have been fully justified for what it has had to offer regarding the mechanism and nature of the process it designates as transference. One of the reasons I have in mind for advocating a further study of hypnotic phenomena is that here is an opportunity for the experimental study of this process. My own feeling is that the transference is the most powerful tool which the physician has at his service for therapeutic purposes, and when we consider that in the vast majority of cases he has not the slightest idea of the existence of this process of which he himself is a part I have perhaps said enough to indicate the importance of its adequate understanding. All forms of therapy, no matter what—surgical, drug, dietary advice, all of them have their component, great or small, of psychotherapy, and the power and efficacy of psychotherapy are bound up in the mechanism of the transference. In addition to this the transference, because it represents a great force, is capable, when used ignorantly, of doing much damage. Under these circumstances it becomes of the utmost importance for the physician to acquaint himself with its meanings, significances, mechanisms, in order that he may make this force available at maximum efficiency for the welfare of his patient. If the time should ever come when the medical profession of this country has to face the possibility of social medicine they should, in my opinion, stand out as a body unanimously committed to the preservation of that relationship between physician and patient which alone makes possible the utilization of this most potent therapeutic force for the maximum benefit of the patient.

The other great movement that grew up alongside the psychoanalytic movement as it developed in this country was the mental hygiene movement. I do not need to dilate upon this to any great extent except to say that it, like its fellow and like other movements generally, was born of intuition, and only after years of growth and development did it become at all clear what it was about or what were its objectives as we know them today. These seem now, in general at least, to be very plain.

To use the language of Whitehead again: "We notice that a great idea in the background of dim consciousness is like a phantom ocean beating upon the shores of human life in successive waves of specialization." [11] The mental hygiene movement is essentially, as it exists today, a public health move-

[11] Whitehead, A. N.: *Adventures of Ideas.* New York. The Macmillan Co. 1933.

ment which has as its major objective the prevention of the disabilities and wastage of mental disease. It has as its goal what I think can best be defined as *the good life,* perhaps qualified by the additional words *well lived.* Its realm is at what I would call the psycho-social level of development, and its methods must be evolved from the basic facts that are contributed by the various sciences which make for the understanding of human behavior. Naturally during the past quarter century psychoanalysis has probably stood first in this contribution. In the last analysis a developed and expanded psychopathology which shall include such well-established principles as come from many directions will be fundamental in developing health programs. Added to this will be a gradually improved technique for getting over the understanding of these principles to the public generally; and from now on the mental hygiene movement will continue to be, as it has been in the past, one of the factors which contribute to that enlarging understanding of the average man which is at the basis of a gradually improving civilization.

Now I will mention another trend which seems to me of outstanding importance, particularly because of the ramifications which emanate from it as a center. I have always said, and I believe, that in the development of scientific thought a new way of thinking is quite as significant and important as the discovery of a new method or a new instrument, and perhaps more so; and herein, in what I am going to mention, we have the basis of a different way of looking at the whole psychiatric field, although the method of thinking seems at first blush to be nothing but the reanimation of something which is ages old. I refer specifically to the work Kretschmer has done on the question of defining certain somatic types and relating to these types certain psychological characteristics. This is perhaps but a new way of dealing with the entire question of constitution, just what I had in mind when I said that this new work was perhaps only a revival of something that was ages old. At any rate, it does involve a consideration of the somatic make-up of the individual, which it is conceded is largely, if not fully, hereditary in origin and which has related with it certain corresponding types of thinking and feeling.

Let me first, before developing the ramifications that issue from a consideration of types, pause to deal briefly with the questions of heredity and environment. Man seems to seek certainty by various devices, some of which inherently lead to erroneous results. One of these devices is the attempt to differentiate clearly, concisely and definitely, when as a matter of fact clear-cut definitions probably exist nowhere in the universe. They are, however, eminently desirable in the wishful attitude that man has toward reality, because they represent definite, conclusive, concrete results of his thinking which he feels are islands of safety that he can rely upon. Unfortunately, however, this aspect of the situation represents only an illusion.

Whitehead says this: "Every intellectual revolution which has ever stirred humanity to greatness has been a passionate protest against inert ideas. Then, alas, with pathetic ignorance of human psychology, it has proceeded by some educational scheme to bind humanity afresh with inert ideas of its own fashioning." Heredity and environment are not any more separate and distinct facts unrelated to each other than are body and mind. Like body and mind, they are two aspects of an organism which grows out of and into an ever-changing environment; and the question as it has been put in other fields is not whether a particular trait is of hereditary or environmental origin, but upon which factor for practical purposes we shall place the emphasis: How much hereditary? How much environmental? we might ask, as Bleuler asked about the psychoses, "To what extent manic-depressive and to what extent schizophrenia?" [12] What really happens in the living organism is that everything is hereditary and everything is environmental, depending upon which facet of the many-faceted crystal of life we may choose to contemplate. Heredity represents the limitations which past experience, as it has been laid

[12] Bleuler, E.: *Text Book of Psychiatry*. New York. The Macmillan Co. 1924.

down in the phylum, imposes upon the growing, developing, evolving organism. Environment represents the possibilities, or their absence, dependent upon the stimuli which may or may not be projected upon the growing organism and result or not in the stimulation of potentialities which are resident therein. It is very important in order to understand the very complex living organism that these dynamic aspects of past experience and present existing stimuli should be borne in mind.[13] Otherwise we lose entirely our possibility of appreciation of the significance of the "temporal coördinate," as it has been called, the "fourth dimension" as it is also named, that is, time as it relates to living things. Now to

[13] For example, certain cases of food sensitiveness, while in their manifestations they definitely seem to be phenomena that are comprised within the frame of reference of chemical dimensions, may on occasion be precipitated by psychological factors which play a sufficiently important part so that they have to be dealt with ultimately in order to secure therapeutic success. This is another instance in which what might be called a constitutional predisposition or an organ inferiority, according to the language which is individually most acceptable, is overwhelmed when subjected to the additional stress of a psychological factor, in this instance a distinct distaste or positive aversion. Under these circumstances one can see that it is possible to have disturbances of various sorts in which the psychological factor plays a greater or a lesser part, according to circumstances, and which therefore appear preponderantly to be physiological or psychogenic in origin.

55

come back to the question of constitution, and you will see why I diverged for a moment to the consideration of heredity and environment, because constitution cannot be understood unless we have this dynamic attitude toward these two aspects of living things. Here in this field we are dealing with largely unknown elements. We can only feel to start with, and because of the principles I have set forth just now, that constitution is not necessarily the fatalistic thing which many consider it. If the dynamic situation as I have outlined it really maintains, then the constitution may be modified, provided it contains latent possibilities of modification and provided it is exposed to adequate stimuli which are capable of changing these possibilities from potential to kinetic.[14] If you will grant me these assumptions, which

[14] The experiments that have been made, particularly in developing organisms, bear out this contention, for it has been demonstrated over and over again that even the genes do not control development absolutely. The cells that would have developed into one structure can be transplanted and so developed into another. For example, if a portion of skin is transplanted to the eye center it is transformed into an eye instead of into skin. The proportion of the sexes in pigeons may be modified by changing their metabolic rate. The large claw of a shrimp may be made to grow on either the right or the left side at will. Many of these changes, at least, seem to be dependent upon certain time relationships and cannot be produced unless the time factor is taken into consideration. In other words, differentiation after it proceeds to a certain point seems to be irreversible, but

A Medical Specialty

I am afraid I may not have made any too clear but which seem to be exceedingly clear in my own thinking, then you will see that the whole question of constitution as raised by Kretschmer's contribution, and those which have come along since and elaborated it, is a question of stage setting, I might call it. It is as if in the drama of life the scenery, the furnishings, the properties, costumes, were all designed in accordance with a certain historical time and place; and upon this stage the life drama is played out and the actions and the words, in short the plot of the play and the way it is developed, must conform with the scenery and the costumes, in other words with the time and the place they represent. There can be no disharmony here or if there is it must be understandable by the audience. Someone may be introduced as an actor who represents another culture, another race, and who therefore is costumed differently and acts differently, but even this discordant note must be consistent within itself. Therefore plays like Julius Caesar, Henry VIII, Catherine the Great, Joan of Arc, and a musical comedy like the Show

at any rate it would appear that the genes are not quite so absolute in their power as has been supposed, otherwise none of these things could happen. Genes, however, appear to have greater possibilities than those ordinarily accorded them and fate seems from this point of view to be less rigidly in control than we had supposed. The possibilities, therefore, of changing so-called constitutional states are suggested by such results,

Boat, are each one consistent with itself in all the various aspects of stage setting, dialogue, etc. No two are alike, no two individuals represented are alike, not even in any one of the plays, but there is no mistaking the significance of the entire production. Time, place, race and culture all fit in in an integrated presentation. And so it is in psychiatry: heredity and environment, somatic structure, psychological function, social significance, cultural forms, all belong together, all are found together, all are related one to another in a consistent, significant way.

This tying together of the many diverse aspects of man as he is studied from the point of view of psychiatry is what I conceive to be the most important contribution of the definition of types which has been essayed from so many quarters these past few years.

Let me elaborate this aspect of the situation a little more definitely in a more specific direction. We have the organicists, who believe that everything, including mental changes, must be explained by some organic background; and we have the functionalists, who do not conceive that any relation to an organic background is essential in their analysis of a functional situation. These two points of view seem to be far apart and I have said in the past that all that we could expect in the future would be that they would get closer and closer together but, like two parallel lines, would never meet. I am not so sure of this position today, but there are certain aspects of this organic-functional splitting, if I may so refer to it, that are of great significance in our present attitude toward psychiatric problems.

In recent work, particularly in the attempt to apply psychotherapeutic techniques to the more malignant psychoses, there has grown up a feeling that there were certain aspects of these conditions which lay beyond the possibilities of being reached by psychotherapeutic methods. In the same way there has never been a clear feeling that we understood how certain psychological states of a very specific character in themselves followed upon certain organic conditions in themselves of a very general nature; all of which leads to the assumption, naturally I think, that there are elements in the symptomatology of the malignant psychoses which extend beyond the limits of what may fairly be conceived to be purely psychological aspects.[15] You see here we are coming back again to something that may easily relate itself, at least in many instances, to constitutional make-up. We are dealing with a possibility that in these serious conditions we may have organic factors, or what I prefer to call biogenetic factors, which lie outside the horizon of the definitely psychological. Such a factor might be, for example, in the manic-depressive group of psychoses

[15] That which occurs in the psyche, however, occurs in accordance with the laws of the psyche.

the factor of periodicity, and such a factor in the dementia precox group of psychoses might be actual deficiencies of cortical cell make-up, or, to more specifically mention a contemporary theory, deficiency for example in the circulatory apparatus which makes the irrigation of the cortical areas by an adequate supply of oxygenated blood deficient, relatively speaking. Of course many other possibilities might be thought of. I am merely mentioning possibilities. Now suppose we do what in fact I am sure has been done in another way with relation to these biogenetic factors and call them general factors. A good illustration would be in the province of epilepsy. As you know, epilepsy has been worked on from all sorts of angles for hundreds of years, and in recent years it has been worked on from the anatomical, the pathological, the biochemical and the psychological angles, and the problem remains unsolved but many things meanwhile have been discovered. The chemistry of epilepsy has been illuminated, the relation of epilepsy to trauma has long been known, the psychology of the epileptic has been a matter of study for years. And yet with all this knowledge and all the possibilities which have been claimed for alleviating the epileptic condition, such for example as are claimed for the treatment by dehydration based upon the theory of that condition and the facts disclosed in its investigation, there nevertheless remains this stubborn fact: that some

60

people receive a cerebral traumatism and it is followed by epileptic convulsions; other people have similar cerebral accidents and no such results follow. Patients who are treated by these advanced methods of treatment are often greatly relieved and improved—the deterioration is arrested, the convulsions are reduced in number—but they continue to have convulsions. To use the everyday language, in such instances the epilepsy is not cured. And so there seems to be some underlying condition which has been referred to as an epileptogenic disposition or make-up, which practically does not mean anything except that such people are epileptics and remain so in spite of anything. Are we not here dealing with a biogenetic factor, a general factor underlying the specific differences as they express themselves in individual cases? We are confronted here with the distinction between bound energy and displaceable energy.[16] The bound energy is that of the more definitely physiological functions; the displaceable, of the psychological. I think it is worth while assuming, as a working hypothesis, that there is such a general factor even though we realize that it does not mean very much when we say it, but it points to the direction in which we must look for further illumination.

It is interesting and significant to point out that

[16] Kardiner, A.: "The Bio-analysis of the Epileptic Reaction." *Psychoanalytic Quarterly,* Vol. I, p. 375.

this way of considering various difficult situations is not confined to the question of epilepsy. We find the same sort of theoretical assumptions in other fields. For example, this is particularly true in the field of mental testing, as especially set forth by the Factor School of psychology under the leadership of Spearman. Intelligence testing generally since the early times has been thought of also in this way. General intelligence, on the one hand, and special abilities, on the other, are what it is sought to test; not that we know really what intelligence is except that it is what is tested by the particular test, but the tests nevertheless serve to classify individuals, perhaps in a somewhat rough but nevertheless measurable way, and it seems fairly evident from the work so far done and the results attained that these tests do as a matter of fact test a general ability, except, of course, for those specially designed tests that are calculated to bring out specific abilities.

I feel of course that this separation of general and special, like all other clear-cut definitions, is an artificiality, just as is the separation of organic from functional; but in our present state of knowledge it is perhaps a useful way of dealing with the material. Naturally we shall continue to hope that these two opposites can ultimately be integrated in a common concept after the fashion of the solution of all such differences.

Perhaps no single concept of present-day psychiatry is so ill-inclusive as that of regression. This is not a new concept by any means but it is, like so many other concepts, an old idea but one which has been so tremendously elaborated in recent years that the difference between the old idea and the new makes the old one hardly recognizable. This concept ties together our whole idea of what might be called the march of life from the past into the present and on into the future, including what I have called the temporal coördinate, involves the aspects of heredity and environment, of general and special, and particularly the concept of differentiation, or, more specifically, individuation as that term has been recently used by Coghill. The fundamental and organic continuum of the living organism is thus considered as a process of unfoldment and differentiation, which process is reversed when regression sets in, and this regression may manifest itself not only in the so-called functional areas but as well in those that are thought of as organic. And so the whole field of mental disease is illuminated and we find ourselves a long distance in advance of the old idea of disease as a concrete entity invading the organism like a pathogenic micro-organism, for example, or of the symptoms of mental disease being something which are expressible by the word "alien." The process of dedifferentiation is one of releasing or uncovering previously developed mechanisms and not a process of addition. It is because of this fact that fundamentally the psychotic pictures with which we are all familiar have so much in common, in fact in many instances could actually be designated as stereotyped. It is on the basis of this mechanism of regression that we can understand such a process as defusion, in which we see instinctual tendencies which had previously been amalgamated and integrated for common ends falling apart, disintegrating, as it were, in this process of regression. In the same way we can understand more thoroughly such a phenomenon as depersonalization, in which the uncovering and outcrop of earlier developed ways of functioning has thrown to the surface material unrecognizable by the host and therefore giving rise to a sense of confusion and unreality. The highly complex, coordinated and integrated pattern of the personality is giving way under the influence of stresses and falling apart in accordance with the pattern of its structure. Expressed from the point of view of the sense of reality, we might say that the patient loses the sharpness of distinction with which he has been able heretofore to separate himself from the rest of the world. Withdrawal from reality, therefore, in this sense, is a withdrawal from contact at higher levels, by which I mean most recently developed and most highly integrated levels, and by virtue of this withdrawal a return to a philogenetically older and more diffuse form of contact. We can see why symp-

A Medical Specialty

tomatology of this kind is so frequent in the early manifestations of mental disorder and how out of the resulting confusion there gradually separate out, by a sort of process of crystallization, certain psychopathic structures. We see this process no more clearly than in instances of individuals who under the influence of an overwhelming emotion commit some terrible crime such as homicide, perhaps killing a person for whom fundamentally they have a profound attachment. Following such an act we find depersonalization symptomatology in evidence for an indefinite time and then we can see the building up of new integrations, which are an effort at cure, let us say, on the one hand, and on the other an effort at avoiding certain too-painful and unendurable realizations. The ramifications of this concept of regression as I have briefly indicated seem to me to be of the greatest use, not only in psychiatry but as a concept in general medicine to illuminate what might be, I think, better called disease processes than diseases.

I believe that we do not as yet know enough to question the organism very fully with regard to the existence, the nature and the operation of some of these factors, the significance of what I have called the biogenetic factors and just exactly their relation to the symptomatology at the psychological level. We have been talking for some years about the organism-as-a-whole, but for the most part this has been a lip service to a concept that I think we all have felt was enormously useful and would in the end produce significant and valuable results; but we have been trained in our thinking for generations to consider the organism as a mosaic of parts, of separate organs and their several functions, and I believe that this talk of the organism-as-a-whole is really only the beginning of a change in our way of thinking, but only a beginning, and it will take probably many years before the concept organism-as-a-whole can really be adequately utilized. We have very little conception, except in the most general sort of way, of the parts that the several organs play in the final total picture represented by the tendencies and directions of the organism-as-a-whole. As I have already mentioned, the recent work on constitution tends to show us how all these separate aspects of the organism can be integrated, how they represent different parts of a large and interrelated whole. But specifically how this works out is another question. What part, for example, does the spleen play in the general orientation of the student's life in his pursuit of the study of medicine? Undoubtedly here is a general factor, more or less obvious. Is there a specific one? Perhaps the time will come when we will recognize in the orchestration of life the occasional notes from the unconscious that will put us on the right track for the solution of some of these subtle and difficult problems.

A Medical Specialty

I can give you perhaps one example that will indicate how I feel such involved questions as this may perhaps be approached. As you will recall, Professor Kraepelin in his great contribution to psychiatry differentiated two major groups of mental disorder: the benign manic-depressive group and the malignant dementia precox group. Then when Kretschmer came along with his types it seemed that the pyknic type belonged with the manic-depressive group and the asthenic type with the dementia precox group. In other words, we have constitutional make-up, types of thinking and character of mental disorder all harmoniously related. How about the pathology of these individuals? Do we find here also a relationship? At the psychopathological level I think it might be fairly said that the manic-depressive group, whatever else we may say about these psychoses, are psychoses of an essentially compensatory character. There is a definite effort in these patients, maintained over a long period of time, to recover their balance, to get well. On the other hand, with the dementia precox group the tendency is quite the opposite. Here is a tendency for the disorder to progress, to become chronic, or in fact in many cases to get worse. The former group might properly be considered as reacting by a process of compensation, the latter group as reacting by a process of decompensation. Now when we come to an analysis of the tissue pathology in these groups we find similar indications. The manic-depressive individual presents tissue changes which show definite tendencies at compensatory types of reaction, while on the other hand the dementia precox group shows equally definite tendencies in the direction of decompensatory types of reaction. For example, in the manic-depressive group we find a considerable percentage of carcinomas, chronic streptococcus infections and circulatory disorders, all of which show compensatory types of tissue changes; while in the dementia precox group we find an overwhelming percentage of active tuberculosis, a material number of cases of death from intestinal catastrophes and acute infections. Tissue changes in this realm of pathology are of the decompensatory type. The picture here is on the whole fairly clear and gives one very definitely the impression that here in the field of pathology we have another bit of confirmatory evidence of the unity of the organism in all of its several aspects, and that if we knew sufficiently how to follow out this concept we would find it carried along into the details of each organ function. Here we are in a field much broader than that of psychiatry. We are in the field of biology, which in its mechanism transcends such details as the psychoses or even mental content at a specific time. We are in a region beyond psychiatry, the understanding of which, however, is becoming increasingly important as we begin to realize that much of our material represents special examples of the general principles here involved.

Nothing perhaps is more characteristic of present-day psychiatry than this tendency toward the unification of what had before been discrete concepts referable to separate aspects or parts of the organism-as-a-whole; and as you know, this general concept has been carried, not so much by the psychiatrists, to be sure, but by others, into the larger field of social relations. I have on my desk, for example, a history of the development of civilization in its various forms, written from the point of view of the influence of the emotions in bringing about these various forms; and I need only call your attention to Spengler's work, which may or may not be considered sound but which does very definitely carry out this point of view, in that he attributes to each culture, to each civilization, to each nation, institutions, practices, organizations—political, religious and social, all of which taken together create a harmonious picture of interrelatedness. Two of the most outstanding examples of the interrelatedness of which I have been speaking, manifesting itself in the organism at both the somatic and psychological levels, are the two very important disease processes known as encephalitis lethargica and general paralysis. In both of these instances both somatic and psychic symptomatology are not only in evidence but are so obvious that each disease might as well be spoken of as a psychosis or as a somatosis. For some reason paresis has generally been considered as a psychosis, whereas encephalitis is generally regarded as a somatosis. In any event, psychic and somatic in both of these instances are so intimately related that they are the natural places in which to seek for correspondences in these two spheres of organismic expression. Both have yielded important results. Encephalitis has yielded its results more especially on the somatic side and paresis on the psychic side, although there are correlations in both instances.

One of the most significant pieces of work that has been done in this country, and one of the most hopeful and illuminating in this difficult territory, is the work that L. Pierce Clark [17] did with his defectives, especially those who had severe organic disease such as epilepsy and hemiplegia. Here he has demonstrated the significance of the psychological component and has made it clear that this factor has to be dealt with in order that the individual may be brought to such a state as to make the best use of his remaining assets.

These considerations, for the most part, have to do with the field considered under the term "constitutional," but there are the organically conditioned psychotic reactions which cannot properly be called

[17] Clark, L. Pierce: *Nature and Treatment of Amentia.* Baltimore. William Wood & Co. 1933.

constitutional but which are the result of the disease process itself, which is organic in nature. The most obvious of these organic situations are the cerebral traumas, and the less obvious are certain symptoms which occur in the course of the psychoses about which there is still considerable discussion as to whether they are properly considered as psychogenic or functional in origin or as to whether they have an organic basis. In all of these conditions it would appear that the clue at the psychological level that we are dealing with organic situations is the impersonal or contentless character of the symptomatology. These indications to my mind mean that the fundamental structuralizations are involved rather than the more superficial patterns which have been constructed at the psychological level and as a result of the individual's personal experiences. Schilder's admirable analysis of psychic disturbances following head injuries [18] would indicate that the main features of this organic symptomatology are the impersonal features at the psychic level, the monotonous excitement, the irritability, the failure in the field of perception and the marked impairment of the Gestalt function. Let me mention some other features that seem to me on the same principle to be of organic import: the periodical fluctuations in the cyclothymic

[18] Schilder, Paul: "Psychic Disturbances After Head Injuries." *Amer. Jr. of Psychiatry,* Vol. 91, No. 1, July 1934. P. 155.

situations;[19] the pyramiding of the delusions, as I call it, in the paretic, which results in the final appearance of delusions of grandeur far exceeding anything found elsewhere and as I believe conditioned by the effort at compensating for a progressive cerebral deterioration of organic nature;[20] the contentless complaints of fatigue or of incapacity for sustained effort; certain memory defects in which the content forgotten is permanently beyond recall; the mechanism of compensation, at least in certain of its reaches. All of these conditions seem to be definitely associated with what we may properly call the

[19] Richter, Curt P.: "A Biological Approach to Manic-Depressive Insanity." Chapter XXVIII of *Manic-Depressive Psychosis*. Association for Research in Nervous and Mental Disease. Baltimore. The Williams & Wilkins Co. 1931.

[20] Similarly with the phenomena of epilepsy, the repeated profound and malignant regression of the seizure is followed each time by what may be conceived as an effort at cure by the utilization of the symbolism of rebirth, which indefinitely repeats itself in its effort to overcome the impossible organic basis of the disease process through the method of reconstitution and rehabilitation of the personality pattern along what may be called normal acceptable lines, and which as it were says each time, "Now perhaps everything will come out all right"; again, as I have indicated that the periodicity of the manic-depressive may have organic foundations, we are confronted by another somewhat similar situation, in which the patient in his several attacks repeatedly attempts to overcome his organically-founded disabilities.

organic.[21] Some of them, however, may be used by the patient for his purposes in a way that indicates, at first blush at least, that they are psychogenic in origin. For example, the fatigue of an adrenalopathy, associated with which is a considerable insurance premium for total disability, may present a picture which seems to be a purely psychogenic affair. The situation is somewhat more complicated, however, in some other instances. For example, in a severe case of dysmenorrhea described by Edwards [22] a physical examination disclosed an infantile type of uterus and a psychological examination disclosed certain marital stresses due to fear of conception. The dysmenorrhea had not put in its appearance before and Crookshank made the suggestive comment that the inferior organ functioned satisfactorily until it was confronted with the additional psychological stress. It is to be regretted that the work on organ inferiority has not been followed up more in detail. It would seem that there are many places

[21] Perhaps some of the more stereotyped symptoms of dementia precox, those that are encountered in the same superficial form in case after case, may depend upon components which are well along on the road to structuralization and are therefore organic in nature. Such a symptom would be, for example, the Egyptian attitude. See my "Language of Schizophrenia." *Arch. Neurol. and Psychiatry,* Vol. 16, October 1926.

[22] Edwards, F. Margery: *Brit. Jr. Medical Psychology,* Vol. 14, Part 2, p. 156.

where the point of view would be useful, especially in connection with the energic concept.

A more definite separation of those psychological symptoms, on the one hand, which are caused by organic conditions, and, on the other, which are purely psychogenic, is very much to be desired. In passing I might indicate that those which are of organic origin, to my mind, may easily become of very great interest and importance, inasmuch as they may represent those features of psychological symptomatology to which more accurate methods of mensuration may be applied more readily than to the definitely psychogenic features. Failures in the field of perception have back of them, for example, a large body of information about the special sense organs and methods of testing and experiment which might easily be applied. As you know, perhaps, I have always felt especial interest in utilization of the energy concept in the field of psychiatry, and it is perhaps for that reason that these matters intrigue me.

To sum up this rather complex statement in a few words, I believe that it would be of great practical significance to make a distinction in our thinking between process and content, and to realize that they may be separately considered. At least in the present state of our information, it would probably be a bootless procedure to attempt by analysis to explain

74

such of the symptoms as I have indicated are largely, at least, of organic origin.

You will note that all through the field, not only as I have thus far discussed it but in many other instances that you can think of, there is this constantly recurring principle of duality represented by the concepts "body and mind," "organic and functional," and in many other ways. I have said that the concept "organism-as-a-whole" would do away with these distinctions, and I have intimated that the distinctions—organic versus functional, body versus mind, general versus special—might be among those that would be thus affected. I have further indicated that the way in which such diametrically opposed concepts are finally discarded is by the resolution of their conflicting tendencies in a concept that includes both of them and thus resolves the conflict between them. Is there such a possibility of resolution in sight? I think there is. I think that if we bear in mind and utilize in place of these disparate terms the concept "purposes of the organism" we will find as we proceed with it that such conflicting terms as "body" and "mind," for example, will progressively cease to be useful. The purposes of the organism are as well displayed at what we have called the organic level as at the psychological, and the terms that are applied to those purposes, such as "compensation," are equally applicable in either field in which they are used. Under these circumstances, you see, we can begin to really feel that the concept organism-as-a-whole is coming to function in a really creative way and to disperse, at least for the present, many obstacles in our thinking created by ambivalencies which have been expressed and laid down in our language. I think you can see the value of this concept in the illustrations that I have used.

I have already indicated that the field of psychiatry is broadening enormously, particularly as it contacts every other department of medicine, and especially as the so-called "organic" and so-called "functional" aspects of disease are less clearly differentiated as our knowledge expands. Anoxemia, for example, locally conditioned by vascular spasm, has been considered the precipitating factor of the epileptic convulsion and later on of the deterioration of this disease, which is based upon actual cellular destruction. Anoxemia of a less violent degree but more continuous has also been considered as basically important in understanding the symptomatology of dementia precox; and here instead of being due to local vascular spasms it has been claimed that the fundamental anomaly was a poorly developed, inadequate and abnormally small heart, which reflected itself of necessity in a correspondingly smaller size of the entire vascular tree. Here are abundant problems for research. Immediate questions suggest themselves with reference to the study of such states as fatigue, and particularly to the study of the psy-

A Medical Specialty

chology of the state of anaesthesia with special reference to the evaluation of the psychological state of
the patient approaching operation, as this may bear
upon the subsequent development of psychotic post-
operative types of reaction, some of which, unfortunately, are malignant in type.

Another very important subject for study because
of its many significant implications is the more intensive analysis of the mechanisms by which patients
spontaneously recover. A patient of mine, for example, under the influence of a psychotic delusional
distortion of his environment, killed both of his
children. This act of his was followed by a condition
of depersonalization which gradually emerged into
a state of clear consciousness, with the exception that
he was hallucinated and heard the voices of his children. They were telling him that they were glad that
he had done as he had because they were in Heaven
and were very happy. Here we have a type of compensatory mechanism with which we are familiar.
Now the interesting part of this man's story as it has
developed to date is that these hallucinations are
becoming less and less in evidence, but his dreams,
as it were, are picking up and taking hold of his
necessity for compensation and they are all pleasant
—dreams of being at home with his children engaged in all the homely joys of family life. Here we
have a transposition from a psychotic reaction to a
definite dream state, which had no socially significant

implications but which is merely a private concern of his own and which would not preclude a possible diagnosis of recovery. How much do we actually know about the mechanisms which are represented by this sort of situation? And if we knew more would it not be possible not only to be more helpful therapeutically but to avoid doing many things which now add fuel to the flames of the psychosis?

To give an example of some very specific possibilities for the utilization of psychiatric technique in general medicine, I would refer merely by their statement to certain formulations that I have made of principles which should be taken into account in the field of surgery. The first of these principles runs as follows: that *an organ or a function about which the important creative aspects of the personality have been nucleated and through which they have been expressed should always be protected with the greatest care and should never be sacrificed under any circumstances, if it can possibly be avoided, for the salvaging of an organ or a function of lesser significance.* The second principle is: that *no operation of election on an erogenous zone should ever be performed unless the patient is psychologically prepared.*

Not only are the psychological factors in disease of significance, but, naturally, we cannot have gone thus far in our concept of the human organism without realizing that there are psychological factors

78

A Medical Specialty

concealed, as it were, in every human reaction. It will probably for some time be the province of psychiatry to uncover these hidden motives. What, for example, are the psychological factors that are involved in the birth control movement, in the sterilization movement, in fact in every significant attitude which man assumes towards himself, towards his fellows, towards the world at large? Thus you see that psychiatry as a medical specialty, at first the problem only of the asylum physician, gradually breaks the bonds of this restricted position and takes up its work alongside the other medical specialties in the office of the extra-mural practitioner. Then of necessity, dealing as it does with the motives of men, it is forced into a consideration of these motives wherever found; and thus it expands, whether the physician will or not, to include an ever-increasing body of thought of wider and wider significance. Some of these implications are of primary social significance.

In closing this lecture let me recapitulate very briefly some of the most outstanding features in the development of psychiatry during the present century as I see them. (a) In the first place and more significant than anything else, it seems to me, is the development of a dynamic in place of a static concept. I can best illustrate this by saying that our language has changed in this respect by the substitution of a consideration of things, organs, tissues, descriptions, classifications, by the consideration of events, processes, relations, meanings, purposes. The moment we have done this we have ceased to think of fixed conditions and we are perforce involved in a way of thinking that commands us to the extent that we think only of processes and relations and aspects of the organism. The fourth dimension of time necessarily enters into our considerations and we realize in a way which we never have before the significance of this factor. We are no longer required to reduce our concepts of a given situation to lower terms, by which I mean that mental facts have meanings in their own right and that they do not have to be reduced to chemical reactions or tissue changes in order to have an understanding of them, although a wider acquaintance with the organism-as-a-whole will result in correlations of this kind which will become of increasing significance. (b) The understanding of mental disease as a process which uncovers already existing mechanisms rather than a process of addition. (c) The development of the concept of transference as one of the most significant and valuable tools for therapeutic purposes which the physician possesses. (d) The integration of all such concepts which have grown out of our study of disordered minds with all the other aspects of human thinking, feeling and acting. (e) And, finally, the understanding of the human organism as reacting at each moment of its existence, not just in accordance with the information which we can gather at the conscious level but with the precipitates of its entire past. In all of these ways we are broadening and deepening our understanding of man in his various activities and expressions, and by so doing improving our comprehension of him when he develops those various difficulties or maladjustments which are known as diseases. In this way it seems to me that psychiatry, without probably any such conscious objective, is working slowly and definitely and surely in the direction of the modification of medical thought—let us confine it to that region—which is nothing short of revolutionary in character, so that an entirely different medical mind is slowly being born, one capable probably for the first time of seeing, at least rationally, as opposed to intuitively, the organism in all its significant meanings unfolding itself at all its levels of activity, in relation to itself and in relation to the rest of the world, a concept which has advanced us a long way from the days of concrete disease entities involving circumscribed areas in specific organs and disturbing their functions and their structures in limited ways which are observable to the laboratorian by means of his various techniques. Such results have only been the beginnings of medicine. The future presents possibilities so vast that I am sure no one would be rash enough to attempt to predict them, and I may add—the methodologies of yesterday will not suffice for the new era.

Psychiatry in its broader reaches and its newer developments, while a strictly medical specialty, has become much more than that designation has ever heretofore meant. The methods that have been developed by general medicine, the emphasis on disease entities, special organs and restricted functions, are being superseded by a new and developing methodology. No longer are the circumscribed observations of the internist, of the clinical pathologist, or the specialized training of the general nurse or even the social worker adequate. We must build a new structure on these new foundations. Tinkering with the old will be but a makeshift. The medicine of the future will be a much more highly evolved and differentiated art than medicine as we have known it.

II

THE SOCIAL SIGNIFICANCE
OF PSYCHIATRY

THE SOCIAL SIGNIFICANCE of mental disease has
been gradually forcing itself upon our attention for
many years, particularly because of the increasing
expense of the care of the mentally ill incident to the
rapidly rising population of our public hospitals all
out of proportion to the corresponding increase in
the general population. From the year 1880 to the
year 1920 the general population increased, in round
numbers, 110 per cent, and the population of the mentally ill in our public institutions 468 per cent. Translated into dollars this meant a corresponding increase
in the budgets of the several States and of the Fed-
eral Government, and, as so often happens, it was
particularly this budgetary increase that attracted
attention to the situation. It was Dr. Salmon who,
shortly before his death, became very much inter-

ested in this question of the expectancy of mental disease and made an attempt to discover the proportion of the population that found its way into hospitals for mental disease in the course of a generation. He tried to find the answer to this question by comparing the deaths in a single year in the New York State Hospitals with those in the general population, and he found that in a given year 1 death in every 22 of those reported to the New York State Health Department occurred in hospitals for mental patients. Comparing the deaths in these hospitals with the admissions, he found that there were approximately twice as many admissions as deaths and concluded from this that 1 out of every 10 or 11 persons became mentally ill in the course of a generation, an estimate which was proved by later careful investigations to be much too high. These later investigations, conducted by Dr. Pollock, Statistician of the New York State Department of Mental Hygiene, and his associate, Dr. Malsberg, showed that, roughly speaking, at the time of Dr. Salmon's inquiry the crude data gave the proportion of those becoming mentally ill in the course of a generation as approximately 1 in 25 or in round numbers 4 per cent. The whole study of this situation gave the expectation of mental disease of New York State per 100 persons alive and sane at specified ages, and showed that the expectation at birth of males exceeds that of females, being 4.7 for the former and 4.4

for the latter. These figures increase to a maximum at the age of 15 years, being 5.5 for males and 5.1 for females, and in the succeeding years there is a steady decrease. From the same study the rates of mental disease in New York State per hundred thousand of the same age and sex, when reduced to the form of a graph, showed the characteristic curve which had been known to us for a long time, namely: a rapid rise during the adolescent and pre-senile and senile periods. At birth, according to all of these figures, the expectancy is in very close agreement with Salmon's rate of 1 to 20 or 22 which he discovered by examining the death certificates, and certainly gives a picture which without correctives would be appalling. To quote from the language of the study referred to: "It appears that approximately 4.5 per cent of the persons born in the State of New York may, under existing conditions, be expected to succumb to mental disease of one form or another, and become patients in hospitals for mental disease. In other words, on the average, approximately one person out of twenty-two becomes a patient in a hospital for mental disease during the lifetime of a generation."[1] This is the situation which has caused and is still causing so much concern. It represents an amount of loss to the community, not only

[1] Pollock, Horatio M., and Malsberg, Benjamin: "Expectation of Mental Disease." *Psychiatric Quarterly,* October 1928.

financial loss but loss in efficiency and in the services of so many people that the mere statement of the case is enough to insure the agreement that we are dealing with a social situation of the utmost significance and importance.

Statistics of this sort, of course, need the most careful interpretation in order that what they really mean may be adequately appreciated and understood. It is to be remembered that we had no statistics of mental disease in this country prior to 1880 and that our statistics have improved materially since that time, and that some increase in the number of patients included in the statistical surveys may be due to that fact. It is also true that the various public hospitals throughout the country have improved their methods of care and treatment so obviously that their reputation has improved accordingly and they are held in much greater confidence by the community. Therefore they are sought much oftener than heretofore. This undoubtedly accounts for a further proportion of the increase. On the other hand, during these years the country has become more thickly populated, great cities have grown greater, new cities have come into existence, and the various social factors that are incident to this increasing population have themselves added still further to an explanation of the increase of mental disease. This increasing concentration of the population is shown by the relative proportion of rural and urban

86

Social Significance

populations during this period. In 1880 the urban population was 28.6 per cent as against a rural population of 71.4 per cent, while in 1920 the urban population had increased to 51.4 per cent and the rural population had dropped to 48.6 per cent, a shift from rural to urban of about 25 per cent of the population. Inasmuch as mental disease which gets into public institutions by due process of law is designated in legal terminology as "insanity," we can understand how this shift of population has had its influence in increasing the number of individuals in public institutions, because we can understand that peculiarities of conduct can be indulged in quite freely in a sparsely settled district which would excite great apprehension and lead to complaints to the proper public officials if they occurred in the congested areas of a great city. These are some, at least, of the artificial reasons, as they might be called, for the statistical increase in the number of patients in our public institutions.

In a study of this statistical situation I wish to call your attention to one set of facts that seem to me to be of great importance, and the existence of which appears to me to have gone almost entirely without recognition. I refer to comparative death rates as between the so-called insane, on the one hand, and comparable age and sex groups of the general registration area of the United States, on the other. The figures are quite startling, as well as significant. They show that the death rates per thousand in the general population in accordance with the age groups that correspond generally with those in public institutions for the "insane," give a total of 13.1, whereas the death rates per thousand under treatment, by age groups, among patients in institutions for mental disease in the United States, show a total of 74.2, or nearly six times as many—to be exact, 5.67 times as many. And if we examine this situation still further we find if we arrange our psychoses in their order, beginning first with paranoia, then the manic-depressive group, then the precox, then the epileptic, and following with the various grades of mental defect—morons, imbeciles and idiots, that there is a gradual increase in the death rate as we go from the top to the bottom. With the paranoia group the age at death is approximately the average death age for the general population, with the manic-depressive group the age at death is a little lower, with the precox group still lower, with the epileptic again lower. Correspondingly, with the morons, the imbeciles and the idiots, it is lower and lower and lower. So that the death rate can be said to correspond with the malignancy of the psychosis as the psychosis is measured from the point of view of capacity for social adjustment. Those who are capable of making social adjustments live as long as the average individual. Those who are incapable of making any adjustments at all, like the idiots, if

Social Significance

they were not cared for would die of starvation and neglect in a few days; under the best conditions of institution life their lives are very short—about ten years only on the average. We see from this situation, therefore, that all that group of varying and varied mental conditions that are classed together under the legal term "insanity" represent disabilities of a character which have a very definite lethal tendency, a distinct, and according to their malignancy proportionate, effect upon the length of life. In other words "insanity," so called, if we wish to consider it in this global way, tends to materially shorten life; and I think it must be obvious to those who are familiar particularly with the malignant forms that it tends in this direction because it interferes not only with social adaptations as such, but even when those adaptations can be made, as in the lucid intervals of the manic-depressive psychosis, it interferes with the continuity of those adaptations, and one of the elements of success in life is just this capacity for continuity.

These facts as I have cited them raise many issues of significance and importance with reference to the relation of the individual to his community, the social significance of his individual conduct and the social significance of mental disorder. The first thing that comes to mind when one attempts to consider these problems is the obvious analogy that exists between the individual of a social group and the component cellular parts of a living organism. We have, as has been pointed out many times, similar forces operating. Individuals, quite similarly to cells, unite for common purposes, on the one hand, while on the other they preserve certain aspects of their individual lives more or less intact. There is from the simple cellular structure to the complicated cellular organism, just as there is from the individual to the social group, a series of increased complications of structure, which complications are produced by a continuous process of differentiation. The cells and the individuals, as the structure grows in size, continue their cooperative arrangements, but they also begin quite early in the process to differentiate so that cells and individuals are set apart here and there for special, peculiar functions which minister to the common purposes of the organism. You see we are approaching again the problems which we mentioned in the last lecture, of the general and the specific, but we are dealing with them here at what might be called a different level, or, to use another terminology, we are dealing with them in a different dimension. The principle, however, is the same, and it is based upon a certain formula which I may express in this way: When two individuals, be they cells or organisms, unite for a common purpose—let them be two men, A and B, who come together in a partnership for carrying on some sort of business—the union of A and B in such a partnership is not ex-

Social Significance

pressible by adding A and B together and setting down the formula accordingly. There is something else that has come into the picture besides A and B— a third component, and that third component is the relationship between them. That relationship cannot be expressed in the formula representing merely the sum of A plus B. So A plus B by coming together in this union have created something, as it were, something new, something which I am afraid we cannot measure to suit our mathematically-minded friends, something which we shall have to classify with the intangibles but something which nevertheless is quite as real as are A and B. Here is a simple expression of the doctrine of emergent evolution. The relationship which has been established by A and B by this coming together is, in the language of this doctrine of evolution, an "emergent." So that the final formula would be, if we reduce A and B to numbers instead of letters: 1 plus 1 does not equal 2, but it equals 2 plus, that is, 2 with something in addition, to which, at the present day, at least, we are unable to assign a definite value.

Now all of this has great significance in my mind as representing a point of view. As I have always held, the way of looking at a thing, the way of thinking about it, is quite as important for purposes of advancing our knowledge as are new instruments or new techniques. Here we are relating the individual to society just as before I get through I shall attempt to relate the different parts of the individual to the organism-as-a-whole, and to call to your attention the very important and outstanding fact that the whole realm of psychiatry lies in the realm of just such intangibles as I have outlined here. Intangibles and emergents are the field in which we function; and the important thing here, perhaps, is to realize that from this point of view, which seems to me to be the correct way of looking at the facts, we begin to realize that the eternal conflict between the organicist and the functionalist really has no meaning, that no adequate explanation of the higher can ever be reached in terms of the lower, because the higher contains the lower and the reverse is not true. My illustration is that while it is true that we never could explain the purpose that lay in the mind of the blacksmith as he pounded his anvil by any examination of the cellular components of his voluntary muscles, it is also true that we could not have a full understanding of how that purpose could be brought to pass without such information. So the necessity of a final understanding of the lower by interpreting it in the terms of the higher—in other words, an understanding of the specific functions of the individual and of the body cell in terms of the purposes of the organism, whether it be society or the individual, is essential if we are going to see these problems in all their dimensions. Nevertheless the understanding of the lower, for example, in the instance cited, the understanding of the structure of muscle, is essential to an understanding of the way in which these purposes are brought to pass.

With this rather tedious, and I am afraid somewhat philosophical discussion, I am brought back to a consideration of what mental disease means in terms that have social significance. Mental disease means, from a social point of view, social maladjustments, and social maladjustments cannot be understood adequately unless we know something of the structure and functions of the individual, just as it is necessary to understand the histology and physiology of the muscle of the blacksmith's arm in order that we might know what was the significance of his failure to perform his functions as a blacksmith as a result of an inability to use his muscles for the purposes of his trade.

We have learned in the individual psychology of the neuroses and the psychoses that the most general cause of these disturbances was what is generally called "intrapsychic conflict," whether this conflict is brought about by tensions between the different aspects of the psychic structure, those that have been described, for example, under the names of the Id, the Ego and the Super-Ego, or whether, on the other hand, those conflicts have been brought to the surface by certain organic inadequacies of the various systems of organs of the body which interfere with expression through these means. At any rate, speaking in terms of energy distribution, what happens in all of these conditions is states of tension produced by frustration. Interferences with self-expression, in other words, result in the piling up of discontents and antagonisms which lead in their turn to unhappiness, inefficiency and maladjustment, on the one hand, or on the other to explosions of a neurotic or psychotic nature, as the piled-up energies that fail to find an outlet through the regular channels provided for their expression short-circuit, as it were, and are expressed in diffuse discharges rather than along definitely provided channels.

In the past, how have these various forms of maladjustment been dealt with? In the early days, of course, they were not dealt with at all in the sense in which they are at present; that is, governments paid little or no attention to them. This is so today in some countries, particularly in the Orient, where maladjusted individuals are permitted to work out their own salvation or destruction, as the case may be. The question of responsibility in such cases does not arise as it does with us. People who for any reason cannot make the grade as prescribed by society have to fall down and take the consequences. If they do things that are taboo the verdict of the herd is thumbs down, without any prolonged inquiry into their mental state or responsibility. But as society advances along the road of differentiation, as great urban centers of population grow, as individuals come more closely in contact with their fellows in these centers of population, departures from ordinary forms of conduct attract more attention, and, what is more important, excite apprehension and fear, and the individuals responsible are extracted as it were from the herd and segregated in hospitals. This method of dealing with these social problems by segregation of this sort has now been going on for some time, and our public institutions have increased enormously as a result both in number and in size. Commitment to the public institution for the "insane" is now a recognized method of procedure.

From these considerations it seems implicit that mental disorder must be understood not only from the point of view of intrapsychic conflict but as measured against the cultural background of the group of which the individual is a part. Of course these two statements are but the opposite sides of the same thing. The intrapsychic conflict is dependent upon the introjected cultural pattern as translated to the individual by his parents and his parent surrogates, and social maladjustment is the expression of the conflict of the individual with the cultural pattern as it exists objectively in his social milieu. Further indication of these considerations is that the same germ plasm maturing under the influence of one cultural environment may result in an individual highly efficient and well adjusted, and in another cultural environment the same germ plasm potentials may produce quite the opposite result; so that, for all practical purposes, at any rate, the effect of a change in the cultural pattern as it may affect individuals is unpredictable, a conclusion which I think has been illustrated over and over again in recent social changes.[2]

The net result of the hospitalization of those that are sufficiently maladjusted to meet the requirements of the law as laid down in the several jurisdictions, is, along with many other factors, playing its part in increasing our understanding of mental disorder, and also of the so-called normal mind. Maladjustments that would never have been called that a few years ago are beginning to be recognized, not only for what they are but because they represent the early stages of more serious involvement, and because in their early stages they can sometimes be successfully dealt with so as to either postpone or prevent the more serious later developments. The trend is definitely in the direction of prevention but we nevertheless still have a constantly increasing load of socially malignant problems for which the only method of procedure which meets the situation is commitment to a public institution. The constantly increasing budget for dealing with this problem in this way is

[2] Mead, Margaret: "The Use of Primitive Material in the Study of Personality." *Character and Personality,* Vol. III, No. 1, September 1934.

one of the important reasons why I think that perhaps the not very distant future may easily bring
significant changes in our program. There is no more
powerful force in society than the force exercised by
economic pressure, and it may be that this will be the
outstanding reason which will appear to alter our
methods of procedure in the future.

As a matter of fact, we are already beginning to
see indications of a changed method of dealing with
this problem. In the first place, we have built up
clinics all over this country to deal with the early
manifestations of mental disease. We have built psychopathic hospitals for dealing with acute mental
disorder, and in most instances they are associated
with medical colleges so that the medical student
may become acquainted with the manifestations of
mental disorder and succeeding generations of physicians will become increasingly competent to deal with
psychiatric and neurotic problems. We have built up
child guidance institutes so that mental disorder may
be recognized in those incipient disorders of child
behavior, in school and out, and the child be set upon
the right path at this time. The prison system is
undergoing a slow but a very definite modification
in its methods by attempting, at least, to deal more
intelligently with the psychotic and psychopathic
types in its population, and by parole, social service
and follow-up attempting to deal with the social
aspects of the problems and help each discharged

prisoner or parolee to maintain himself in lucrative and socially useful occupation. These are some of the things that are happening, but certain other things are happening, too. Psychiatry may easily come in for its share of consideration in accordance with methods which once prevailed more largely than they do now and which have been taken up by other departments of medicine. I refer to the method of dealing with the patient in his home so long as that is possible, rather than bringing him to a hospital. This, as you know, was the method in many places in Europe, of which Gheel, in Belgium, is perhaps the best known example. It is a method which is now represented in general medicine by the visiting nurse; and in order that it should be applied in the field of psychiatry it will be necessary that the apprehension and the fear of the mentally ill individual in the public mind should be allayed. In other words, to put it very briefly, it is to my mind quite possible, at least in selected and appropriate communities, to undertake the care of mentally ill patients in their own homes, and to remove to hospitals only people who are very seriously sick or dangerous to themselves or others. In fact this plan is already in operation to some extent—I have not full information about it —in Australia, and its advantages are obvious in saving an enormous amount of expenditure for capital investment in huge institutions which, like everything else that is built in this rapidly-moving age, at best soon become antiquated and out of date. Obviously a plan of this sort, however, cannot become effective in any large way until the average physician and the average nurse and the average social worker are much more highly trained in the symptoms and the care of the mentally ill than they are at present; but I think it is fair to say that this state of affairs is coming to pass with a reasonable degree of rapidity. And so I am suggesting that this may possibly be one of the ways in which a solution of this enormously important social problem may be attempted.

The socialization of the feebleminded might take a similar though somewhat different course. I am thinking more particularly of the possibility of industrializing this group. Whether and when this can be done will depend almost entirely, I think, on the capacity of employers to appreciate their limitations and their place. There is no inherent reason why groups of feebleminded should not render good service in the more or less routine, stereotyped activities of factory life, and enjoy it. Under these circumstances it would be necessary, however, in order to protect them and the community, that they should be taken care of much as we take care of them in our hospitals. They could be housed in villages under the supervision and care of trained personnel and could be made very effective workers who, under these circumstances, would be infinitely happier than if left to their own devices to be preyed upon by the

99

unregenerate members of the general community who are always looking for opportunities of this sort. Such methods, without being dignified by especial social recognition as such, are actually incorporated in the practices of certain European countries where more or less defective children are set aside for the simpler tasks, the girls to do the housework, the boys to do the labor on the farm.

In connection with this whole matter of the hospitalization of the so-called insane, the matter of medical education needs to be borne in mind. The advisability and the importance of modifying the medical curriculum along the lines of the increasing number of hours devoted to psychiatry has been long under consideration, but with the realization that 50 per cent of the hospital beds throughout the country were mental beds [8] and with the increasing de-

[8] The following analysis reduces the situation to units of hospital days, as follows:

Total hospital days in United
   States in 1933 = 296,000,000 total

   _____

   173,000,000 mental *
   85,000,000 general
   22,000,000 tuberculosis
   16,000,000 other special hospitals

   _____

   30,000,000 more patient days in
1933 than in 1929 in mental hospitals.

   * Including feeblemindedness and epilepsy; excluding them, 146,000,000.

mand upon the part of the public for psychiatric service the medical colleges have yielded to the result of surveys and recommendations and are pretty generally responding to the needs of the situation. The medical student is being exposed to a very much more prolonged contact with psychiatry, the exposure begins earlier in the course and before he has made up his mind what specialty he wishes to pursue; and this increased importance of psychiatry in the curriculum of the medical college is also being carried over to the curricula in the nursing schools and in the schools for social workers. So that we are developing quite rapidly now a very greatly enlarged personnel who have some knowledge and understanding of mental mechanisms as they are found outside of institutions, in the family, in the office, by the social worker, in fact everywhere. Now to add to what I have said about the family treatment, particularly of acute mental illness or mild mental disturbances, this picture of a growing trained personnel, it can be seen that when the doctor and the nurse and the social worker know as much about Susan with the "vapors" as they do now about Tommy with the stomach ache, then we will be in a position, perhaps, to realize a program developed along the lines suggested. All these suggestions have in mind the criticism which has long been implied and often expressed in the attitude of relatives but is now, it seems to me, coming at least a little more to the front and with somewhat more authority, namely, a criticism addressed against the institutions for mental disease and which in the main claims, as is also claimed of hospitals for somatic disease, that there are certain disadvantages in accumulating many people similarly affected together, treating them more or less *en masse* in an atmosphere in which their difficulties may be mutually reënforced by contact with their associates. I will not dilate upon this criticism further than to say that I believe that it has a certain cogency and justice and to add that some of the defects which are pointed out by the critics are capable of being met in an adequately administered institution. There is, however, a serious criticism addressed against the stigma which the institution places upon the individual, and this, I am convinced, remains a reality in spite of everything that has been said to the contrary; and this stigma is enhanced and made more definite by the stupid, cruel, archaic and unnecessary legal procedures which surround hospitalization.

With regard to this whole matter I think I can best quote certain excerpts from the Report of the Royal Commission on Lunacy and Mental Disorder,[4]

[4] Report of the Royal Commission on Lunacy and Mental Disorder. Presented to Parliament by Command of His Majesty. London. His Majesty's Stationery Office, 1926.

made in 1926. Among other things it states as follows:

The commission was appointed—

"(1) To enquire as regards England and Wales into the existing law and administrative machinery in connection with the certification, detention, and care of persons who are or are alleged to be of unsound mind.

"(2) To consider as regards England and Wales the extent to which provision is or should be made for the treatment without certification of persons suffering from mental disorder.

"And to make recommendations."

Here are some extracts from the Report:

"The modern conception calls for the eradication of old-established prejudices and a complete revision of the attitude of society in the matter of its duty to the mentally afflicted" (p. 16).

"The keynote of the past has been detention; the keynote of the future should be prevention and treatment" (p. 17).

"Contrary to the accepted canons of preventive medicine, the mental patient is not admissible to most of the institutions provided for his treatment until his disease has progressed so far that he has become a certifiable lunatic. Then and then only is he eligible for treatment. It is, perhaps, not remarkable in these circumstances that the percentage of recoveries in public mental hospitals is low. In our view the position should be precisely reversed. Certification should be the last resort in treatment, not the prerequisite of treatment (pp. 18-19).

"It is remarkable that in the case of a form of disease probably more subtle and difficult of diagnosis than any other, the layman should insist on his right to sit in judgment on the expert" (p. 20).

"If the true conception of a mental patient is that he is suffering from an illness, we cannot help feeling that those who desire the further elaboration of legal machinery are apt to lose sight of the common sense of the matter" (p. 20).

"The problem of insanity is essentially a public health problem to be dealt with on modern public health lines. So only will the atmosphere of suspicion and aversion with which the subject is invested be dissipated" (p. 22).

In commenting upon the report of the Royal Commission a London correspondent says:

"Every facility should be afforded to the mentally ailing to submit voluntarily to treatment; but when compulsory detention is unavoidable, the intervention of the law should be as unobtrusive as possible."

Social Significance

These recommendations, as they are involved in the foregoing statements, seem to me to be very little to expect of our legislative bodies; and when we realize that the march towards a better understanding and treatment of mental afflictions is dependent upon so many factors, and that this after all is only one and perhaps in some respects an unimportant one, then surely reforms along these lines should be demanded by an enlightened public opinion.

In any event, the hospitals have not yet exhausted their possibilities for helping the patient, and if this new method of outpatient treatment ever does come into being it will overlap the present methods of hospital care. Hospital care has opportunities for improvement in several directions. Perhaps the two most significant are a greater understanding and utilization of inter-human relations which would enable us more adequately to classify our patients, not only with relation to each other but with relation to the hospital personnel, and a still further enlightenment regarding the mechanisms of recovery so that the various agencies of the hospital could be more intelligently addressed to assisting these mechanisms than they frequently are at present. Then, too, it would be wonderfully encouraging if the principle of research could be recognized so that every appropriation for new hospital buildings would automatically allocate one or two per cent for purposes of research. This would be a really forward-seeing development.

At this point it seems to me that the most significant aspect of the social relations of psychiatry to be discussed is the mental hygiene movement. This movement, as you know, had its inception in the activities of Mr. Clifford W. Beers and its official birth by the formation of the Connecticut Society in 1908. In the short space of a quarter of a century it has spread over the entire civilized world, having branches in practically every country. This most stupendous growth was concretely illustrated by the First International Congress on Mental Hygiene, held in Washington in 1930. It is doubtful if any movement for the betterment of health has ever spread with such rapidity and been accepted in principle by such a large body of people throughout the world. Its original objectives were simple humanitarian ones that had to do with a concerted effort to improve the care of the "insane." This rapidly spread to include the feebleminded and then the criminal classes, by which time it had grown to large proportions, developed high ideals, and was well launched upon its course as a major public health issue. Now it is essentially a movement which has as its principal objective the prevention of mental illness, which involves its recognition long before it finds its way to the state hospital. In carrying out this program it is interested in making practical ap-

plication of the developments in the fields of psychotherapy and psychopathology, and in general in
coming to an understanding of human beings that
will make it possible to work out a practical program
not only of prevention but of the road to follow that
will lead to the finest results in living. It is interested in all research work which will add information that is utilizable for these ends and furnish
tools to assist in their carrying on. It has profited
very largely by the contributions of the psychoanalytic group to the understanding of human conduct, and much of the mental hygiene work is done
under the banner of psychoanalytic concepts, at least
the more generally accepted ones. You are all, I am
sure, sufficiently well acquainted with activities in
these lines so that they need no special illustration
by me. I will add only one thought at this point
which seems to me to explain the rapid growth of
this movement. It has been generally conceded for
some time that mental hygiene, and, for that matter,
psychiatry, was oversold, but whether the reasons
for this state of affairs are generally appreciated I
do not know. My own feeling is very decidedly that
the reason is simply this: that people without knowing very much about either mental hygiene or psychiatry look upon them almost as they might a
saviour come particularly to ease them of their bur-
dens. People apply to the psychiatrist and the mental
hygienist for every conceivable reason, and the ready

acceptance of this movement is to my mind based upon the wishful thinking of the masses, who want to have some help and encouragement to struggle through a burdensome life in a cruel world. They would like to have it, too, by way of the methods of magic. If they could only be cured by the laying on of hands or the recital of a cryptic formula they would be tremendously satisfied. And so in their helplessness and their distress they look to this new movement as a promise of assistance; and I am afraid that in many instances the protagonists of the movement have often made promises that have encouraged such hopes. Of course we have a right to look to the future with optimism, but we cannot expect to attain our goals by magic. We have to work for long years to bring to pass what we even now feel to be fairly well-established goals. This is by no means said in discouragement, for I do not feel discouraged. On the contrary, I feel that a tremendous amount has been accomplished and if the future looks discouraging it is only because the present has been so brilliantly illuminated that we see not a few but a multitude of things which are indicated to be done.

One of the outstanding results of the mental hygiene movement has been to call attention to the practical advantages of introducing psychiatric concepts in various situations. The early efforts that were addressed to the improvement of the care of the "insane" naturally led to an effort to find out something about the patients who finally landed in the state hospitals. This resulted in an effort at getting at etiological factors, with the resulting improvement and elaboration of case histories and case studies. The factors that came to the fore as a result of these studies demonstrated that the patient who arrived at the state hospital was not an acutely sick person in the same sense that a patient with pneumonia is acutely ill, but that as a matter of fact he was suffering from a condition which had had many years of incubation and which at the moment of his arrival at the state hospital was already, in most instances at least, an end result of a chronic process. These conclusions were in harmony with the psychoanalytic school that traced all mental illness to the first five or six years of life. As a result of the conviction of the importance of these early years there came about the movement to overtake, as it were, mental illness in its growth, and psychiatrists were sent into the universities and into the schools, where these conditions were known to develop. And then finally the whole subject of education became a matter of psychiatric interest and is so still. Whether changing methods of education can eliminate some of the factors which we feel now to be at the bottom of a great deal of serious mental disorder later in life is one of the fascinating fields for present exploration.

Twentieth Century Psychiatry

Similarly this method has branched out in the field of criminology, where it is struggling with the problem of so-called crime. Here it meets with antiquated, outworn, archaic ways of thinking that have been crystallized in the statutory law and retain personal expression through the personalities of the lawyers who have been educated in the traditional legal methodology. Nevertheless psychiatry is making its impression and the law schools are gradually, if slowly, responding to the pressure of a slowly-evolving public opinion; and the old-fashioned theological concept of sin which now interferes so seriously with any intelligent functioning of the state in these matters of social maladjustment which are known as crimes is gradually getting out of the picture, and the day seems to be coming when these conditions will be treated purely from the standpoint of what the best results are which can be hoped for and what the best methods are of obtaining them, with the idea of salvaging as much of the human material and of the wastage incidental to the maladjustments as possible. Such a point of view eliminates entirely the idea of punishment, as I believe it should. If this could be done then the welfare of the individual and the welfare of the state could be given judicial and adequate consideration, and the program of dealing with the individual offender elaborated accordingly. As it is now, the process often exacts a greater toll of suffering from the innocent family than it does from the culprit himself, and the stigma which falls upon them all because of the delinquency of one is quite of the same nature in many respects as the stigma of mental disease. The future, it is hoped, will bring that degree of enlightenment which will lift this burden from so many who now suffer it, for it will be understood, for example, that a particular arrangement of genes in the germ plasm is totally out of the control of anyone and therefore is something for which no one is responsible. A recent author has given the possible germ plasm combinations in an average human mating as five million billions,[5] so that any particular individual might be said to have been the result of one of these combinations. The absurdity of attempting to hold anybody responsible for the results that are expressed in figures of such magnitude is obvious. The same thing might be said of the practically infinite objective situations into which this unique individual is projected during his lifetime. Attempt as we will to control reproduction in the direction of eugenic results and to modify environmental influences during the growth of the individual, it is obvious that failure must take place in a certain proportion of instances; and that these failures should be hated and punished and killed, that they should be held to be wicked and sinful and stamped with the social

[5] Stockard, Charles R.: *The Physical Basis of Personality*. New York. W. W. Norton & Co., Inc.

stigma of a special class, from which not only they but everybody related to them also suffers, and that this should all be done at the expense of everyone concerned, representing liabilities of untold extent, presents a picture which it will be, I hope, one of the accomplishments of psychiatry to modify in the direction of a sweet reasonableness and a deeper understanding. And the crowning absurdities of this whole situation—and I say this not critically but only emphatically, for I am sufficiently familiar with the way in which these practices and concepts developed to have some understanding of them and therefore to realize that they are not absurdities except in the sense in which I now use the term as over against our concepts which we have developed in recent years about man and his ways of thinking and acting—the crowning absurdities, as I say, are the hypothetical question and the question of responsibility. The question of responsibility is entirely a philosophical one which no one can answer. The hypothetical question asks something about an individual who does not exist, never has existed, and from the constitution of most of such questions never could exist. It is in harmony with the entire criminal procedure, which does not try the defendant but tries a hypothetical individual accused of something the existence of which often is questionable except by definition. The trial that takes place in our criminal courts is not the trial of a man but the trial of a ghost that stalks across the stage in this dramatic procedure and that probably would be least recognized by the so-called criminal himself, while behind such indefinable terms as "responsible" there hides the same old motive of vengeance. The attempts and the failures that man makes to protect himself from himself are nowhere shown clearer than in the field of criminology. Nowhere, therefore, is the help of the psychiatrist more needed. The following is a quotation from Professor Perkins, Professor of Law at the University of Iowa, and indicates an effort at a practical improvement of the situation along lines which are possible in the face of existing legal and social traditions: "The effort of the Classical School to establish in advance an exact measure of punishment for each transgression, by the creation of new offenses, and the division of others into degrees, etc., has been found to be inadequate. The modern trend is toward individualization of treatment as evidenced by such techniques as indeterminate sentence, probation and parole. Unsoundness of mind of every kind and degree would seem to require consideration in a fully developed scheme of individualized sociopenal treatment; but it would seem wiser to leave most of this field to the part of the machinery which functions after conviction, than to inject an increasing amount of it into the jury trial itself. Probably the social interests in the general security and the social interests in the individual life would both be promoted by

keeping within rather narrow limits the kind and
degree of mental disorder which entitles the defendant to a verdict of not guilty, while at the same time
readjusting the machinery after the point of conviction in such a manner as to keep abreast of every
contribution of science in the field of disorders of the
mind." [6]

[6] (This footnote is cited by Professor Perkins in his
article on Partial Insanity in the *Journal of Criminal
Law and Criminology,* Vol. XXV, No. 2, July-August,
1934.)

"The following committees met in joint session in the
Mayflower Hotel, Washington, D. C., May 11, 1934:
American Psychiatric Association—
    Dr. William A. White, Washington, D. C.
    Dr. V. C. Branham, Albany, New York.
    Dr. Winfred Overholser, Boston, Massachusetts.
    Dr. C. P. Oberndorf, New York City.
American Medical Association—
    Dr. William C. Woodward, Chicago, Illinois.
    Dr. Winfred Overholser, Boston, Massachusetts.
New York Academy of Medicine—
    Dr. Israel Strauss, New York City.
    Dr. Dudley D. Schoenfeld, New York City.
American Bar Association, Criminal Law Section—
    Mr. Louis S. Cohane, Detroit, Michigan.
    Mr. Rollin M. Perkins, Iowa City, Iowa.

"At this meeting it was unanimously agreed that it is
desirable to keep within rather narrow limits the kind
and degree of mental disorder which will entitle the
defendant in a criminal case to an acquittal and to re-
adjust the machinery after the point of conviction to
the end that mental disorder which is not sufficient for

Social Significance

Some of the immediate problems relating to crime present important research possibilities. It is very important to know, for example, how far the criminal, so called, is restricted and confined to anti-social methods of conduct, first, by the forces with which he comes into the world as a result of a peculiar and unique combination of germ plasm genes, and, secondly, how far his conduct is modified by the quite usual vicious environment in which he grows up; and,

an acquittal may result in treatment other than that provided for persons who are not mentally disordered. After some debate, it was also agreed by all that for the present it will be better to formulate statements of principle along these lines rather than to attempt at this time to draft proposed legislation. Thereupon certain statements of principle were prepared, including the following which received the unanimous approval of those present:

1. Criminal incapacity by reason of mental disorder should be limited within very narrow bounds. The end to be achieved is to have only the most extreme cases of mental disorder recognized as grounds for acquittal.

2. A defendant acquitted on the ground of insanity shall be committed as a matter of course to the appropriate state hospital for mental diseases; subject to release only on conditions applicable to the release of other committed inmates of the institution together with the approval of the trial court or other appropriate tribunal.

3. Provision should be made whereby mental disorder which is not sufficient for an acquittal may result in treatment other than that provided for convicted persons who are not mentally disordered."

more specifically, it is important to know the nature of these forces as they operate on his Super-Ego systems. In terms of energy questions are easily formulated, such as, Are his excursions into anti-social conduct the result of an unusually strong libido drive or are they the result of an exceptionally weak Super-Ego control, or do both of these factors play into the situation, at least in many cases? And what, if any, is the nature of other dynamic, intrapsychic mechanisms, and how are these related to so-called constitutional traits which may be expressed in bodily structure and function? To revert to the problem of typology as it presents in these days: the principle of indeterminacy, as laid down by Heisenberg, is to the effect that position and velocity cannot both be measured at the same time. If position is determined velocity cannot be, and if velocity is determined position cannot be defined. A recent writer has translated this principle in psychology by saying, "We cannot predict if we measure, and we cannot measure if we predict." [7] By measurement he means quantitative determinations which do not include the time element in accordance with the methods of the physics of yesterday, whereas a constantly changing system presents difficulties that are not capable of being met by such methods. Accurate measurements

[7] Shuey, Herbert: "Recent Trends in Science and the Development of Modern Typology." *Psychological Review.* May 1934.

of the kind indicated are applicable in the dead-house, not to the living individual. We must therefore be exceedingly careful of the results that are claimed by various measurements now in use, and realize that, apart at least from the criticism just indicated, these measurements are only of parts of the organism, from which it is exceedingly dangerous to reason to the whole. However, the principle, as it seems, may include a self-defeating element. Now typology does not undertake static measurements but defines a type in much the same way as so-called disease entities are defined, and undertakes to indicate the direction in which such types develop. If the writer I have just quoted is correct, the success attained in prediction of the future development of types will be in inverse proportion to the capacity for applying detailed measurements to them of a static variety, as I have indicated. The principle involved is, "That any system in motion or change cannot be measured accurately without changing or stopping this motion or change." [8] In this way we get a new concept with which to deal, and as the type involves the organism-as-a-whole it contains all the factors essential to prediction as far as these can be considered without reference to the play of forces upon them, but these factors then of necessity elude accurate measurement. Here we are involved not only in a highly controversial but an extremely in-

[8] Shuey: *Op. cit.*

tricate development in the field of psychology and psychopathology. I mention it because I think it significant and important and one which will probably play an increasing part in future developments. Its special importance at the moment lies in the fact that it is a movement which tends to counteract the confidence which we have acquired in recent years in our various psychological testing schemes, particularly the intelligence tests. Testing intelligence gives us a static concept of just where the individual stands at that particular time, but it gives us no information about the direction in which his energies are moving, which is in many respects much the most important thing to know about an individual.

Another important aspect of the question of typology, and perhaps a part of the same situation I have just discussed, is the statistical study of the distribution of types. It is to be noted that quite characteristically these distributions result in symmetrical, bell-shaped curves showing the minimum number of extremes and the maximum number of means. It is questionable in my mind whether such curves are actually informative as to the objective realities to which they refer or whether, on the other hand, they are not projections of our mental attitudes toward these realities.[9] Of course this really

[9] *The Biology of the Individual.* See discussion at end of Chapter IX, "Constitutional Aspects of Personality Types," by Eugen Kahn. Vol. XIV of the Research

Social Significance

must be so. The only question is, How much is it so? and whether man by any method can escape in part or altogether from the limitations of being himself a part of that which he undertakes to understand and measure.

One of the important results in typology has been to disclose the fact that different types are incapable of understanding each other. The classical example is that of the introverted and extraverted types. Two such individuals in their language use the same words but what each says is incomprehensible to the other. The whole point of view, the whole orientation of the personality, is different in each instance, and if we are to understand individuals we must most assuredly take account of these differences.

The attitude toward crime and the criminal classes is perhaps the most outstanding example which could be chosen of man's prejudiced feelings about himself and the incorporation of these prejudices into his thinking and acting. Man has from the very beginning thought very well of himself. His early concepts of the universe were that the sun, moon and stars were put into the heavens in order that they might light and warm him particularly, that the sun revolved about the earth, the earth because it was the habitation of man being the center of the universe and man being the flower of creation was the par-

Publications of the Association for Research in Nervous and Mental Disease.

119

ticular object of the love and consideration of God. This tendency has always existed. It is a part of man's feeling of insecurity and what I have called the safety motive of his thinking, his feeling and his acting. He seeks safety and security in such beliefs, and he resists, and always has, anything that runs to the contrary. He has been inclined, probably because of his laziness, to believe that his instincts were absolutely correct guides to his conduct and that common sense was all that was necessary to insure success in this life. In the face of repeated examples of failure of instinctive processes and the inadequacies of common sense, his feeling of insecurity is activated and he resists the evidence of his senses. In the same way he has disregarded the evidences of his inadequacies which come from the emotional side of his life. He has regarded himself as having reached the peak of evolution and presenting innumerable perfections, at least in their possibilities, but he has failed to recognize the disrupting and death-dealing tendencies that run along side by side with his greatest possibilities. And so in dealing with criminals he has exalted his own feelings of perfection at the expense of others' mistakes and blunders, has characterized them as sinful and bad, and by implication considered himself, by comparison at least, as good and therefore worthy.

This same attitude has crept into the educational system, the whole scheme of the relationship between teachers and students and unfortunately, too, between parents and children; and education has unfortunately had as its main objective the compressing into a common mold of all the varied possibilities which the individual child represents rather than an effort to discover in each one his outstanding capacities and to enable him to unfold all of those marvelous qualities with which he has been endowed and develop his capacity for living to the fullest possible extent. Experimental efforts, of course, have been made in this direction, but the swing from an undue rigidity of standards to their complete absence has been from one extreme to the other, and there has been little appreciation of the value of striking a happy mean whereby the individual might be considered from the point of view of a social unit. As such, society becomes of absolute importance to him, as only through it can he find his greatest individual development, and, *per contra,* only through the greatest individual development of each unit can society reach its greatest possibilities. Education of the individual and development of social standards are mutually related in this way and must be considered, not apart, but together. It is but another instance of the organism-as-a-whole versus the separate parts considered by themselves.

From a consideration of all these various aspects of psychiatry as it has developed in this and that direction it seems obvious that it is altering our viewpoint about human beings so profoundly that this changed viewpoint is coming to be a definite and important and significant part of the cultural pattern into which future generations are to be born. The new point of view as it unfolds and develops will therefore have as the years go on an increasingly important modifying function with relation to our knowledge of ourselves and our feelings towards others, and should have a definite tendency to knit the individual social units together into a more coherent and integrated whole that will function at the social level more effectively and at least with less obvious lost motion.

When all physicians know as much about the general principles underlying psychiatric thought as they do about the general principles underlying other medical specialties, they will see their patients from this angle as well as from the somatic angle and changes will begin to happen in the relation of patient and physician and in the treatment of the patient which it would seem must have far-reaching results. The fundamental character of these results will become more apparent as the same sort of knowledge spreads to the nurse and to the hospital administrator. Further than that, the point of view for which psychiatry stands will seep in every direction through the social structure, so that hereafter it is conceivable that wherever human adjustments are involved there will be someone to voice the principles that have been uncovered by psychiatric thought and demand for them an adequate hearing. If this day is delayed it will only be because progress in this new, and what we call the psychiatric point of view, has been slow in finding its way into our educational institutions other than the medical colleges and the universities. It is as important that instruction should be carried on in accordance with mental hygiene principles in the early years as it is to expose medical students to psychiatry early in the course of their education; and it is as important that the teachers in the primary schools should know something of the principles of child behavior as it is important that heads of hospitals, prisons, industrial establishments and other great collections of human beings should understand something of the material with which they are dealing and the laws by which it is governed. It is true that at the present time we have a great deal of experimental educational procedures in various types of schools, but the whole huge educational machine is too unwieldy and too ponderous to be rapidly influenced or materially changed in a short space of time. The change will come slowly; and it is perhaps desirable that all of these various changes that I have indicated should come at the tempo which would enable them to relate themselves to each other adequately instead of one group outdistancing another and thereby for that very reason adding stresses unnecessarily.

Twentieth Century Psychiatry

Perhaps one of the next developments of social significance in psychiatric thought will be a definite recognition that there is a psychology of interhuman relations. Up to the present time psychiatry has largely been a medical specialty, and as such was interested in dealing with the sick individual. Therefore its point of view has been addressed more particularly to the individual, and such efforts at social amelioration as have been undertaken have been undertaken from the standpoint of correcting individual maladjustments. In the field of industry, for example, it has been obvious in recent years, when competition has become progressively more acute, that the employer could no longer afford to spend six, eight, ten months or more in giving an employe an opportunity to learn something by experience which perhaps he never could learn, and at the end of that time dismiss him because of incompetency. This expressed an amount of lost motion which keen competition made it necessary to look to as a source of waste. On the other hand, it is equally evident that to deal with an individual employe in this way did not give him a fair chance. And so all such matters are now beginning to be seen from the standpoint of adjustability or the contrary of an individual for a given job, in his own interest and in the interest of employer equally. Of course industrial psychiatry has many ramifications other than this, but this illustrates what I have in mind; that is, that

Social Significance

social conditions have been approached mostly from the individualistic standpoint. Now if our comparisons and analogies with living organisms are correct we may be sure that a social structure represents a higher form of organization than the individual structure, that as such it presents new and more complex forms of relationship, and therefore that the psychology of the individual can never be a complete answer to the psychology of the group any more than the physiology of the single cell can ever be fully competent to explain the entire multicellular organism. It is for this and similar reasons that I believe that one of the next steps will be the recognition that there is a field for psychology and psychiatry in interhuman relations which will be best approached, not from the individualistic point of view, but with the appreciation that we are here dealing with a higher integration, and with a group of manifestations which both hang together sufficiently and are enough different from others to constitute a special scientific discipline of their own. It is easy enough to speculate upon the stupendous possibilities which might result from the development of such a new department of thought. Communities small and large, municipalities, states, nations, would come in for their respective consideration; and there might easily come as a net result principles of international relationship of the utmost significance to a world constituted as it is today by being knit together by means of communications that are gradually welding it into closer relationships in spite of the maintenance of widely diverging interests in many respects. The human organisms in its social relations would thus call for understanding in these, its broadest activities, and it is by no means out of the question to conceive that its activities might even under these circumstances be reduced to principles and laws.

For example, as I write these words I have on my desk before me a work entitled, *Emotion as the Basis of Civilization,*[10] which undertakes to define the outstanding cultures from the point of view of the emotional patterns which they evidence. It would appear that the cement substance of society, the cohering forces that keep masses of people together acting in uniformity, consecrated to common purposes, is by no means intellectual in nature but is predominantly emotional. While I think that most of us would agree with this statement, I have the feeling that while the emphasis on the emotions has been an exceedingly valuable one, nevertheless we are a little inclined to take the distinction between intellect and emotion somewhat too literally. We forget our prime concept of the organism-as-a-whole and are led by the seductions of language into a consideration of the intellect and the emotions as if they were

[10] Denison, T. H.: *Emotion as the Basis of Civilization.* New York and London. Charles Scribner's Sons. 1928.

two separate mental processes instead of being two ways in which for our convenience we look at mental processes; for I do believe that they can no more be separated than can mind and body, and that what we would actually find if we investigated the matter more deeply would be that wherever we have what is apparently an emotional situation that the intellectual aspects of mind would be relatively little in evidence and *vice versa,* but that the two would always be distinguishable, and when we have for example relatively primitive emotions ruling the day those aspects of intellectual action which we can see in the situation will be also relatively primitive. For example, one of our paranoid patients of some years ago had spent practically a lifetime in running away from his persecutors. It seems that he had an invention which enabled him in his opinion to extract gold from sea water, and his persecutors were after him to get the invention away from him. This projection mechanism operating in this way is a comparatively primitive type of psychological reaction. It involves factors that we see in the animistic period of culture among savages. Now if we look at the intellectual aspect of this individual we discover that that, too, is equally primitive. His idea of getting gold from sea water was to sail the ocean in a vessel with a paddle wheel in the center arranged with buckets which dipped up the sea water, which ran in a sluice over electro-magnetic plates, and that the electrical attraction for the metal would extract it from the sea water—a plan which would be altogether too silly and primitive for any schoolboy to entertain.

At this point, if time and space permitted, it would be appropriate to say something about the nature of truth, but I will merely add that it is important to realize not only the qualities that man possesses in common with his fellows but the differences that make him in each instance unique. These differences ensure his living in a world somewhat if only slightly different from that of his fellows, and so truths and facts as we ordinarily know them are modified as they are translated by each individual in accordance with his make-up and past experiences. The psychotic individual illustrates these differences very clearly, and in our social structure we see all the phenomena of ambivalence and of opinions based upon different levels of development which are very helpful in understanding their origin and significance.

From these considerations and with the addition of the fact that I think we must accept, namely, that psychiatry can probably never undertake any adequate plan of treatment for all those who need help, at least according to any of the therapeutic standards that now maintain, it will be evident that the outlook for the future will depend very considerably upon the slow alteration of cultural standards in conformity with our increasing knowledge of the psychology of mental disorder. These standards, if they follow along this development, will probably have the function of easing stresses at weak spots, and more particularly of offering opportunities for self-expression and development in greater abundance than they are offered at present, so that each one in his own character may develop more freely in accordance with his own inventory of assets and liabilities and approximate more nearly maximum possibilities within the limitations that his make-up entails. With the growing appreciation of the significance of the facts of the psychic life, and their subjection to the standards of scientific thought and research, and the fact that in the fields of education, social work, general medicine, and in fact throughout the field of man's activities, they are becoming more and more generally recognized, we are led to feel that we have a right to expect that these cultural changes will take place perhaps along the lines I have indicated. So that we have two great sources of hopefulness in this constantly enlarging field: hopefulness that comes from the expanding therapeutic possibilities and techniques as they are applied to the treatment of individual cases, and the expansion of the horizon of our thought about matters psychiatric as each case adds its mite of information to the general fund of our knowledge; and the incorporation, little by little, of these results in the cultural patterns as they are laid down from generation to generation.

III

THE
GENERAL IMPLICATIONS OF
PSYCHIATRIC THOUGHT

Not so long since, a scientist—I believe he was an astronomer—came out with the statement that now science had advanced to such a point that it was possible to describe the universe. By which he meant that the laws that govern in whirling nebulæ, in the vastnesses of space, as well as the laws that govern the structure of atoms, were all sufficiently known to warrant his statement. That this immense sweep from nebulæ to atom—while no one of course but a fool would claim that all was known about it, still it seemed to him a fair statement to make that no really significant features remained unobserved and that there were no great hiatuses which remained completely unknown. This ambitious statement attracted my attention because, with the tremendous grasp which science has upon the cosmos that could make it possible for this man to make this statement, in making it he did not mention the mind of man. It seems to us who are dealing with the mind difficult to understand how a man of scientific stature sufficient to make such a statement as I have outlined could possibly conceive of the universe without realizing that that conception was itself a function of mind. It is one of those lapses which illustrate how frequently the obvious eludes us. Man seems by preference to think of himself as if he were outside the universe rather than a part of it; and the fact that he is a part of it is one of those things that has to be repeatedly relearned, but it is so important a concept from my point of view that this process of re-learning will have to be repeated sufficiently often until it becomes a part of our permanent equipment. In any case it seems fairly obvious that no one could undertake a description of the universe without realizing that this description is part and parcel of man's observation of the universe and takes the form dictated by his special necessities and interests. The form of the universe, in other words, as it appears to man is necessarily a function of his mind. If there is any doubt of the truth of this statement consider how different a world must be that of the person who has been congenitally deprived of a special sense such as sight or hearing, and how different the world must appear to the new-born child and how the world grows and develops parallel to the growth and development of the special sense organs and perception. The mind, like the camera obscura, reflects a certain aspect of the universe in miniature; and so it may be said, I think with propriety, that the world within and the world without are so related to each other that they exist like the opposites day and night. Each one has its particular form and content only because of the other. This philosophy is not new. It is a way of thinking which in some form or other has intrigued man for many centuries but it is rather interesting to see that psychiatry throws some light on this situation, in fact that certain phenomena with which we are familiar tend to further this way of thinking about the cosmos. I call your attention particularly to the nihilistic delusions, to the delusions that certain patients have that the universe is falling down about their shoulders, so to speak, that everything is disintegrating, disappearing, reverting as it were to its original state of chaos, that perhaps they themselves do not really exist. They may, in their own estimation, have died long ago and been buried. You are familiar with the symptoms. The psychoanalytic theory is very helpful—it is that the libido cathexes have been withdrawn from the external world, which, to put it more simply, means that the patient has lost interest in the things that are going on about him, or that in a sense he has actively undertaken the destruction of a hostile world.

General Implications

The significance of this psychotic state of mind seems to me to be that it indicates very clearly how the world within and the world without relate themselves to each other. It has always been conceived that the world within was dependent upon the world without, but here we have definite indications that the reverse is also true. While no one doubts that our perceptions and our ideas would cease to exist if there were nothing to provide stimuli from outside realities, here we have a definite indication that these outside realities would cease to exist if this world within should disintegrate. The two are part and parcel of a reciprocal relationship and, as I have already indicated, neither one can exist without the other. This point of view I think to be so significant that it is fundamental; and its importance is comparable, in my mind, to such events as the substitution of the Ptolemaic conception of the universe by the Copernican, the advent of the Darwinian theory of evolution, Freud's contribution to man's knowledge of himself. I would add this fourth important concept, not only of the relation between the two worlds, that within and that without, and the necessary dependence of one upon the other, but the fact that this is so because man is a part of the cosmos and in the course of evolution he has come into existence by the differentiation of forces which operate upon and within him as they do elsewhere. If the theory of evolution in its larger aspects is true, then life must in some way have come into existence by a process of differentiation and development and evolution from the non-living. Mind in the same way must also have arisen from the forces which in their operation produced life; and as I do not believe that there are any great hiatuses in this progression from inorganic to the highest types of social coöperation based upon ideals, I must necessarily believe that the energies and the forces that operate throughout nature continue to do so in the realm of the psyche, and that they operate in accordance with the same laws there that they do elsewhere. I have expressed this belief elsewhere by saying that it could be formulated in the statement that mind was an environmental inclusion. This conclusion, it seems to me, forces itself upon one who undertakes a comprehensive view of the entire situation.

One of the criteria of the importance and significance of any new point of view or way of thinking is that it fits in with similar new ways of thinking in other relations. It is interesting to note in this connection that Sir James H. Jeans in his Presidential Address to the British Association for the Advancement of Science last year took as his topic "The New World-Picture of Modern Physics," [1] and in that lecture he says, among other things: "There is, in fact, no clear-cut division between the subject and object; they form an indivisible whole which now becomes

[1] *Science,* Vol. 80, No. 2071, Sept. 7, 1934.

nature." And then further, in speaking about the difficulty with which we labor in order to understand what we psychiatrists usually speak of as reality, he says: "It may seem strange, and almost too good to be true, that nature should in the last resort consist of something we can really understand; but there is always the simple solution available that the external world is essentially of the same nature as mental (*sic*) ideas." Sir James designates his position with reference to these recondite questions as one of philosophic idealism. I do not believe the psychiatrist can avoid these philosophical considerations. More and more the world we live in demands in our thinking some comprehensive formulation. The more nearly pluralistic universe of the nineteenth century has given way all along the line to attempts at correlation and integration; and it will depend somewhat upon our philosophical point of view, whether we know it or not, how we look upon some of these problems that reach beyond what might be conceived to be purely the boundaries of psychiatry.

Of course I realize that such a philosophical point of view is essentially deterministic. I do not pretend that I can solve the problem of free will as against determinism, which has vexed the minds of people from the very beginning. But here again psychiatry has a very valuable contribution to make, and the psychoanalysts are those who have brought to us most specifically the importance of the deterministic attitude. Whether determinism rules the universe and all its parts or whether there is something that corresponds to freedom of choice, is a question that probably will be decided by each one according to his temperament. I only know that man relinquishes the idea of freedom very reluctantly. The physicists today are taking up the principle of indetermination but they confine it to phenomena of very small dimensions. They nevertheless seem disposed to hang on to the principle. As to the merits of the case I have no opinion, but I do know this: that unless we acted "as if" we believed in determination we might as well give up the study of psychiatry in its various ramifications. Unless we were convinced that psychological events were preceded by adequate causes which could be determined by sufficient investigation, then we would simply have no objectives toward which to orient ourselves. And we do know that by hewing closely to this attitude of determination we have discovered many things which otherwise would have remained mysteries.

The advent of the principle of indeterminacy disturbed me until I realized that after all it was but a projection of our own way of thinking upon the outside world of events. That being the case we need not expect to have our world destroyed. A working equilibrium would some way be found. We must probably accept the principle that observing a phenomenon in some way changes it. At the present the

issue seems to be whether we are to go on with the
concept of a deterministic universe in the usual sense
or whether we must become resigned to a universe of
statistical probabilities.

In this connection I feel bound to mention the
question of heredity, because the reasoning here runs
parallel to that in relation to determinism. It would
not be difficult to argue that if we accept determinism we must accept the full responsibility of
heredity, and that therefore everything that we do
or think is mapped out beforehand in such a way
that there is no use trying to do anything about it;
and herein lies the danger of an attitude of mind of
this sort. If we believe that everything psychopathological is based upon an hereditary background which
determines in its very inception and for all time what
the consequences shall be, then truly there is nothing
to be done about mental disease at all. Therapy is a
useless and a gratuitous waste of time and we might
as well fold our hands and let the world wag along
without worrying ourselves about the results, or
exerting ourselves to change them. But here we have
exactly the same situation that we had with reference to determinism. We know that if we act "as if"
we could modify human beings, "as if" their difficulties were removable, "as if" they could be cured, so
to speak, of certain disabilities, that it is truly remarkable what extraordinary results are sometimes
obtained. So that both in the field of determinism

137

and that of heredity we must pursue a philosophy of "as if." These are not the only places where "as if" must rule. I have referred previously to the whole subject of mental testing. All sorts of tests have been devised for all sorts of purposes; particularly, and the best known, is the test of intelligence which, as it is now used, is used in the form of the Stanford modification of the Binet-Simon. This test has now been in use for many years and yet if we tried to find out what this intelligence is that we are testing we would find that no one knows. Intelligence up to the present time is indefinable. It is so complex and so intricate that it eludes any effort to compress it into a single formula. This has finally become obvious to the people who are engaged in this work themselves, and so instead of speaking of intelligence they speak of "test intelligence," which is equivalent to saying in response to the question, What is this intelligence that you test?—"It is that which is tested by the intelligence tests." This on the surface seems a rather ridiculous state of affairs. Nevertheless, again we discover that by using these tests we have unearthed an enormous amount of information. We are enabled to classify people in all sorts of ways which are useful to our understanding of them and to our methods of dealing with them. We have here measuring rods which, to be sure, are not accurate in the sense of the physicist and the mathematician, but which are roughly capable of making separations between individuals and groups which are valuable for us in guiding us in our methods of dealing with these individuals and groups. Again we find, therefore, that the doing of things sometimes strangely and almost mysteriously does away with the objections which seem to be insurmountable when the discussion alone of the doing is under way. Plenty of individuals can find reasons for inaction. It is the person who acts who sometimes works the miracle. It was Leonardo who asked, "Is it the caprice of Fate that man must see to know, must be blind to act?" The value of psychometry depends mostly upon the ability of the person who applies it. The result in this field as in others is on this account often superior to the tool or the method used.

If we would understand the human organism, and particularly the human mind, from the point of view made possible by present-day psychiatry, we must realize that we will have to change our thinking processes completely. In fact we will have to change them in a way that amounts to a complete about-face from the way in which we were accustomed to think a generation ago.

The old structural academic psychology assumed that on the psychological side the finished product, the idea for example, could be traced back to its elemental constituents, which in this instance were sensations. The sensation was the unit of psychic structure and the psychic state at any particular moment was a mosaic of such sensations, very much as one might conceive a bit of matter to be a mosaic of molecules. Similarly the nervous system was constructed of units. In this case the unit was the reflex, and the complicated processes of the higher centers were but the mathematical summaries of reflex arcs. During the present century, however, these views have been slowly changing. The study of child psychology, for example, has demonstrated that the child does not acquire first a series of discrete sensations and then put them together so as to form perceptions, so that these perceptions are nothing more nor less than the sum of the sensations which compose them. This limiting mechanistic hypothesis has been headed for the discard for some time and is now definitely in the waste-basket. The child's first experiences are not of such a nature. The first experiences are comparable, using a biological analogy, to the protoplasm which is the basic substance of life. The first experiences of the child are already perceptions, perceptions with respect to which it attempts to relate itself. The difference between these perceptions, as the difference between protoplasm and the higher forms of life, is a difference in differentiation. The specific and the concrete are not amalgamated to make the complex, but out of a relatively homogeneous background these concrete constructs differentiate and emerge; so that development and evolution proceed by a process of differentiation and emergence and it becomes evident that the whole is not expressed in the sum of its parts but the whole is more than the sum of its parts, for by the organization of the parts and their relation to each other something enters the situation which is possessed by none of those parts separately.

This, you will see, is a very different way of looking at nervous and mental patients than the way of a generation ago. It has been particularly brought to our attention in this country by the researches of Coghill, especially his researches on the embryonic forms of *Amblystoma*. In speaking of the results of his investigation of the development of behavior he says: "The behavior pattern from the beginning expands throughout the growing normal animal as a perfectly integrated unit, whereas partial patterns arise within the total pattern and, by a process of individuation, acquire secondarily varying degrees of independence. According to this principle, such an entity as a 'simple reflex' never occurs in the life of the individual; complexity of behavior is not derived by progressive integration of more and more originally discrete units; the conception of chain reflexes as usually presented is not in accord with the actual working of the nervous system. On the other hand, within the total, ever-expanding integrated organism-as-a-whole, partial patterns emerge more or less and tend toward independence and dominance, but, under normal conditions, always remain under the supremacy of the individual as a whole." Here you will see that the process is one of the gradual differentiation, or as he calls it "individuation," of specific movements from the background of the total pattern. Referring to the development of the movements of the appendages of the *Amblystoma,* for example, he says: "As the appendages develop the total pattern expands into them with the result that at first they move only as the trunk moves. A little later they move as part of a postural pattern and take definite positions or attitudes according to the posture of the trunk. Still later the appendages acquire patterns of their own which, when performed in response to a local stimulus, are known as reflexes. Discrete limb movement is therefore acquired by a process of individuation within an expanding total pattern. The process is one of analysis, not of synthesis." This means, as you will see, that the reflex, which we used to think was one of the building blocks of the nervous system, an entity so to speak in itself, never occurs in any such isolated fashion but is "dominated by the total behavior pattern."

You will see that this biological work leads us to two very important and significant conclusions, important and fundamental for psychiatric thinking. One is a reënforcement of what I have already mentioned of the two concepts, the general and the specific, for here we see that a reflex, which we have always thought of as a highly specific type of reaction, never, as it were, separates itself from its background, the total behavior pattern. So that we begin here to get away from mere lip service to the concept of the organism-as-a-whole and discover actual biological reactions of a concrete type which demonstrate the correctness of what is implied in this concept. And, secondly, another principle of equal importance, which the English philosopher Schiller expresses in these words: "Things must be explained by their significance and purpose instead of by their 'causes,' by their ideals instead of by their potentialities," which is but another way of saying what I have referred to when I have called attention to the increasing importance of meanings and values as over above descriptions. This formula, too, is an excellent starting point for what I suspect is going to be a difficult task for many years to come, namely, the knowing how to ask the organism by way of particular experiments and observations the questions which are becoming increasingly more important as to what are its purposes as they are exemplified and illustrated by the functions of its different parts. Let me give an example and you will see the significance of what I am aiming at. In epilepsy we find that the convulsive condition is associated with an alkalosis. Now the convulsive seizure itself, with the violent contractions of the musculature, produces as a result lactic acid, and the lactic acid tends to restore the acid base equilibrium. We see here what for our purposes and for our ends is much better expressed in terms of the purposes of the organism than simply in chemical equations.

One of the outstanding needs of psychiatry is the development of methods for querying the purposes of the organism. The value of such tests as the Rorschach test is that it tests the general pattern of the personality. It is not a test of vision but by means of this highly differentiated function it gains access to the more general pattern. So long as the testing of part functions as taken over from the laboratories of general medicine is expected to unravel the secrets of mental disease we will continue to miss the real point—the characteristics of the general pattern.

This change in the way of thinking about organisms and their functions, and the functions of their parts, and their relations to one another, has found its way into the general concepts of medicine and is beginning to alter materially the physician's viewpoint in many fundamental ways. The mosaic concept of the organism, which sees it built up of separate structures added together, was the outcome of a type of thinking which considered diseases as entities somehow or other involving, implicating or being added to the organism under certain circumstances. Such statements as that of Sydenham, made two centuries ago, that: "A disease, in my opinion, how prejudicial soever its cause may be to the body, is no more than a vigorous effort of Nature to throw off the morbific matter, and thus recover the patient," were forgotten; and, as Dr. Campbell has put it, it seemed as if the average doctor had come to think of his patient as "the more or less incidental container of an interesting biochemical, physiological, or bacteriological situation." We are constantly forgetting that words and formulations and classifications are mere conveniences with which we attempt to reduce to order and to understanding that total mass of experience which must have been for all of us originally, to use the words of William James, "a big, blooming, buzzing confusion." How different a concept from the static, restricted, simplistic, naïve concept that Campbell describes and how diametrically its opposite is that of Peabody, who says: "What is spoken of as a clinical picture is not just a photograph of a man sick in bed. It is an impressionistic painting of a patient surrounded by his home, his work, his relations, his friends, his joys, sorrows, hopes and fears." To have effected this change is to have made enormous progress, but think of the years it has taken. Old ideas die hard, to be sure, but they die much more slowly when they are imbedded in the traditions of our daily living and disguised in our language. Then is it indeed a difficult thing to extract them from their hiding places, bring them out into the open and dissipate their influence by a conscious appreciation of the absurdities for which they stand.

The concept organism-as-a-whole needs further elaboration. I will, however, only briefly mention two aspects of this concept along which elaboration would seem to be needed. In the first place, it is obvious that the process of differentiation involves the creation of emergents, that is, of an organization which, like water, is unlike its constituents, hydrogen and oxygen, and the possibilities of which are not predictable from a knowledge of the characteristics of those constituents. Secondly, let me quote a few words again from Whitehead to indicate my meaning here: "It is the definition of contemporary events that they happen in causal independence of each other. Thus two contemporary occasions are such that neither belongs to the past of the other. The two occasions are not in any direct relation of efficient causation. The vast causal independence of contemporary occasions is the preservative of the elbow-room within the Universe. It provides each actuality with a welcome environment of irresponsibility.... Our claim for freedom is rooted in our relationship to our contemporary environment. Nature does provide a field for independent activities. ...

"The causal independence of contemporary occasions is the ground for the freedom within the Universe. The novelties which face the contemporary world are solved in isolation by the contemporary occasions. There is complete contemporary freedom. It is not true that whatever happens is immediately a condition laid upon everything else. Such a conception of complete mutual determination is an exaggeration of the community of the Universe." [2]

These are two principles that need to be everlastingly in mind. I mention them here because of their importance, and in addition because I think that some of the current misunderstandings are explained by them. For example, I think that one of the reasons why the anthropologists are so hesitant to accept psychoanalytic interpretations is because these principles are not hewn to. Two cultural institutions, religion and marriage for example, may be rooted fundamentally in the same needs, but as they grow by the process of differentiation they develop independently side by side, which is of course not to say that they may not modify each other, but that is very different from being causally dependent one upon the other. These independent modifications have been going on for thousands of years and it is not strange that the anthropologist hesitates to accept interpretations which are derived from the analysis of individual patients. Social and cultural institutions develop as such and according to laws that control them in their evolution quite as definitely as they do

[2] *Adventures of Ideas.*

individual organisms. This is perhaps expressing it a little too strongly, but I think in principle it indicates the nature of the difficulties involved, difficulties which, as we might expect, are by no means inconsiderable.

And thirdly, another principle which perhaps overlaps or includes those already mentioned is involved in this new way of thinking, and if we would understand modern psychiatry it is important that this principle should be clearly in our minds. It is this: We have advanced beyond the point in our thinking where we deal or attempt to deal solely with concrete entities, whether these entities be disease entities, ideas, concepts or what are known as facts. The advance that we have made is that we have come to the point where we realize that dealing with these discrete elements is not enough. In doing so we lose the most significant aspects of the organism. And so we have come to a realization that it is the relations between these elements that are of prime significance. Psychiatric thinking is coming more and more to emphasize this matter of relations and thus to raise the whole quality of our thinking to a higher stage of integration.

Our reliance upon common sense is gradually becoming more tenuous, and the new universe which is being created as the result of scientific advance requires for its understanding the hardest kind of thinking and an open-minded willingness to discard in the process most of the conceptions with which we have been brought up. Even if common sense as a method of procedure, or, to be more technical, even if common sense as a methodology is not to be discarded but still pursued, as it probably will be, nevertheless the material with which common sense must deal undergoes such considerable changes in the course of time that the net result is about the same as if we had concluded to disregard common sense. Anybody in the days of Columbus who had any common sense at all knew perfectly well that the earth was flat. I believe, as a matter of fact, most people believe so today. However that may be, the average school boy in our public schools who studies geography, if he has any common sense at all, knows just as definitely that the earth is round. And so the things that common sense has to take hold of are undergoing constant change in the course of our growth and development. If today we find our common sense quite worthless at assisting us to understand what the physicist means when he speaks of a time-space continuum, we may be pretty sure that the next generation, or at least a future generation, will have as little trouble with a concept such as this as the generation to which we belong has with the concept that the world is round.

I have called your attention to what I often speak of as pseudo-problems: the problem of mind and body, of heredity and environment, of determinism versus free will; and I have implied that these various opposing points of view, like all conflicts, will reach their resolution only in another point of view which includes both of them and which is at a higher level. The body-mind conflict, despite the fact that it is still maintained by ardent controversialists, is becoming less and less significant, less and less important. When we speak as I have of the purposes of the organism, such a concept can be expressed in either so-called organic or so-called functional terms. In fact the difference between functional and organic is perhaps only a difference that can be expressed by the terms reversible and irreversible. If a pathological state can really be undone then it is reversible and the state properly designated as functional. If it cannot be undone then it belongs in the category of the organic. The qualification here naturally is, however, that what cannot be undone today we may find means of undoing tomorrow; and so, like all our other material, it is subject to the everlasting, continuous changes of growth and development, and furthermore, even conditions that are irreversible in the individual may have their results modified as factors in the emergents of culture. We may never find a cure for cancer but our whole attitude towards it and our understanding of it and our feelings about it may be very greatly modified, for example, by a changed attitude toward the whole question of death.

General Implications

This leads me to a brief consideration of an hypothesis which seems to have attracted very little attention in the psychiatric field except by implication here and there. It is the maturation hypothesis. I think that it will be generally conceded that the newer viewpoints in education move in a direction of development in techniques for assisting the growing, developing organism of the child to unfold its greatest possibilities. This of course should be visioned from two sides, namely, the giving to the child an opportunity by removing the inhibiting obstacles in his own make-up, such as bashfulness, doubt and indecision, and placing him in an environment which offers the stimuli which are most conducive to this unfolding process. Thus both education and psychotherapy call upon the inherent forces of the individual, which if unimpeded lead to normal maturation. And, too, in both instances the progress of maturation is furthered by the creation of a situation of safety in which the individual feels free to develop his own personality. In the psychotherapeutic situation this is brought about by the transference of the analytic situation.[8] Of course the two aspects

[8] Coghill speaks of growth as follows: "Growth may be conceived as the creative function of the nervous system, not only with regard to the form of the behavior pattern but also with regard to its control. The creative component of thought, upon this hypothesis, is growth.

"Man is more than the sum of his reflexes, instincts, and immediate reactions of all sorts. He is all these,

frequently, if not always, overlap. I am asking you to think of the problems of psychotherapy from this point of view: Whether it is not helpful to consider that the release of fixations and the overcoming of repressions belong to the freeing of the individual from inner inhibitions, and his change to another environment as having the effect of exposing him to a different set of stimuli? In fact this latter method, the change to another environment, for a long time was almost the only effective tool that those who dealt in the therapy of childhood maladjustments had at their hands; and that it worked extraordinarily well in many instances is of course due to the fact that the child is a very plastic organism, relatively speaking, and could make new adjustments with comparative ease during these early years. Later on this method becomes less certain in its

plus his creative potential for the future.... The real measure of the individual, accordingly, whether lower animal or man, must include the element of growth as a creative power. Man is indeed a mechanism, but he is a mechanism which, within his limitations of life, sensitivity, and growth, is creating and operating himself."

Coghill, G. E.: *Anatomy and the Problems of Behavior*. Cambridge. The University Press. 1929.

The old term "orthogenesis," which for some reason seems to have been discarded, might very well be revived unless the newer term "maturation" really includes the concept which that used to express.

operations;[4] and the psychoanalytic method has been developed largely to deal with those inner difficulties which operate quite as definitely to interfere with development in certain inhibited sectors of the personality.

I believe this concept has value because if it is adequately thought through it will be realized that it involves a larger point of view than the point of view of either heredity or environment, that in fact the restrictive aspects of the heredity-environment point of view are lost in this larger generalization. Every reaction of the organism is both hereditary and environmental. Heredity only takes place in an environment, and development itself is a function of the unfolding organism. Whether we attribute more to heredity and less to environment, or the opposite, is wholly a matter of personal opinion, personal prejudice or individual temperament. Up to the present perhaps we have thought of heredity more especially as presenting certain limitations to the organism. It can as well be thought of also as presenting certain possibilities, the possibilities, however, only to be realized by exposure to the stimuli adequate to their development. In such terms as "instinct," for example, which is the functional

---

[4] The time factor is here important. This has been shown experimentally. Modification is limited to certain early phases of development.

appearance, as it has been assumed, of hereditary tendencies which have been accumulated through the ages because of their survival value, we have almost anthropomorphized our reactions in this regard quite as much as we ever did in the old Faculty Psychology when we spoke of knowing, feeling and willing, as if these could be taken out of their settings and considered separately. It is quite true, to be sure, as Spearman states, that "wholes can no more be studied efficiently without reference to parts, than parts without wholes"; [5] but we cannot use wholes to prove one thing and parts when we want to prove another. We must continuously bear in mind the fact that these various ways of considering organisms are dexterities which we have developed in order that we may manipulate the facts of experience. Quite the opposite point of view of this anthropomorphic instinct with which we have to deal so much in our literature is that developed by Josey, who puts it this way: "Given an organism with a certain structure, physiological condition, and mass of experience in a certain environment, there will be generated out of this situation forces which are as strictly determined as any force generated in the physical world. Outside of such situations there are

[5] Spearman, C.: "The Battle Between 'Intuitionists' and 'Psychometrists.'" *British Jr. of Psychology.* April 1934. (General Section) Vol. XXIV, Part 4.

General Implications

no *forces* affecting the organism and impelling it to various activities or desires." [6]

Such a point of view as this has the advantage, at least, of compelling a consideration of every situation as far as possible free from prejudice, developing its significant meanings on the basis of the actual findings rather than upon hypotheses, such as that of the instincts, which may be more or less nebulous.

Even with such modifications of the instinct hypothesis and the introduction of the maturation concept, we are still at a loss to account for many of the results of psychotherapy and for some of the results that occur spontaneously in the psychoses. Of these spontaneous results I have particularly in mind the rapid changes that occur in the manic-depressive reaction states—the sudden shift from depression to exaltation, the rapid lifting of a depression which has been in existence for a considerable time; and, in the precox group, the equally sudden shifts that take place, the coming out of a stupor and the lifting of a depression in the matter of a few hours that may have been in existence for years. The mechanisms that account for these changes are still a matter of mystery, and both with reference to them and all other processes in the psychoses that make for recovery I believe we have a very fruitful material for research work. The more we know about the way these various conditions get well spontaneously

[6] *The Social Philosophy of Instinct.*

155

the more intelligently we can in our treatment play into the hands of the forces that make for recovery.

To touch upon a subject which is a rather far cry from any of those hitherto considered, I should like to discuss for a few moments in certain of its relations the subject of anxiety. As you know, for many years, in fact ever since the theory of evolution has been a subject of controversy and investigation, the question has constantly reasserted itself as to how evolution is brought about. The general doctrine has long since been accepted by scientific men, but the mechanism of the evolutionary process, the manner in which the processes of life are loaded, as it were, so that they operate in the direction of evolution, has never been satisfactorily solved. At present the production of mutations by radiant energy as it affects the germ plasm seems to be holding the center of the stage, but even here I think there are serious difficulties in the way of adequately explaining the evolutionary process as being initiated in this way. Now while I shall not attempt to solve such a weighty problem as this, still I think that in the same way that the nihilistic delusions threw some light on the relations between the organism and the environment, anxiety will throw some light on the way in which the evolutionary mechanism operates at the psychological level. In the first place, anxiety, as the term is technically used, differs from fear in the sense that fear relates to outside circumstances which

threaten the organism, whereas anxiety is a warning
that there are certain inside conditions which are
developing and which may be destructive in their
effects upon the organism. It is generally conceded,
I think, that anxiety is perhaps not only one of the
most frequent symptoms at the psychological level
but that it perhaps is the most frequent symptom. In
fact by the very matter of its definition one would be
disposed to assume that very few people could go
through life without from time to time experiencing,
if ever so lightly, the symptom of anxiety. It results
when sublimations threaten to fail and repressive
forces are on the verge of being overwhelmed by
instinctual demands. It is an indication that the balance of power within the psychic systems is moving
in the direction of the instinctual processes. Anxiety
itself constitutes an exceedingly painful state of
mind; in fact in its more severe manifestations it is
unendurable and almost any means of escape from
its torment may be chosen by the patient. If you will
get this picture, therefore, you will see that at any
given time when either the instinctual forces are
strengthened or the repressing and sublimating
forces are weakened anxiety may develop, and in
these circumstances one of the solutions that presents to the patient a means of escaping the torment
of this mental state is to do those things which will
reconstitute the supremacy of sublimation and repression, or, in other words, to move in a direction

away from the instinctual forces and towards those processes which make for development in the direction conceded to be evolutionary. If I am correct in this assumption then we may assume, I believe, that anxiety is one, at least, of the outstanding forces which drive man along the path of development and civilization. I should dislike to think that it was the only force, for if that were so then all of man's virtues could be explained by fear. I cannot but believe that while anxiety may be a compelling factor, it should be considered as it were as pushing from behind, whereas other forces which attract from before, in accordance with the ambivalence of all manifestations of energy, need to be fully taken into account.

In conformity with my tendency to think of things in terms of energy, I feel that anxiety, as a danger signal, is apt to be raised when the amount, or to use a more recent physical term, quantum, of libido in repression tends to become excessive. In other words, if sublimations fail or outlets of expression close and so lead to frustration, then libido accumulation threatens the equilibrium of the psychic structures by breaking through and leading to instinct manifestations which are so destructive in their nature as to develop anxiety. It is very interesting in this connection to bear in mind the theory which has been advanced, I believe, from time to time, that civilization and progress are dependent upon repression, and specifically upon the restrictions which have been placed upon the activities of the sex instinct, and that higher cultural developments are reached by a process of what might be called a recapturing of the energy that would otherwise be expended along these channels, and, correspondingly, that a decline of culture is accompanied by the reverse conditions. Naturally the question will arise whether these phenomena are causes or effects. At any rate, they are interesting for consideration along the lines of the accumulation of libido and the development of anxiety, as I have just indicated.[7]

As I have already stated, I believe that practically the same laws govern at the psychological, and from my point of view more particularly the psycho-social level of development, as govern lower down at the physiological level. The comparison of society to an organism, such as Hobbes made in his *Leviathan*, is not to my mind just simply an analogy but is a useful way of looking at the facts of life as they present to us at their different levels of development. Therefore if we think of the social organism as expanding, developing and differentiating just as does a growing organism, and think of anxiety perhaps as a motive force which helps the drive along this pathway, then we may think of psychiatry in

[7] Unwin, J. D.: "Review of Sexual Relations and Human Behavior." *Brit. Jr. of Medical Psychology,* Vol. 14, Part 2, p. 198 ff.

this large scheme of life as making its contribution
to our understanding not only of man's place in nature but of how he functions, what may be expected
of him, how he fits into the general scheme. It seems
that the organism in its development, particularly
that aspect of its development which has indicated
its continued greater elaborateness of differentiation,
is striving, as it were, to contact more and more
aspects of the environment, as if by doing so it continuously came closer to the possibility of mastering
that environment. It is a process to which the living
organism seems to be doomed in perpetuity, and it is
a process which it seems of necessity must always
fail. Forward the organism develops in response to
this inherent urge, always seeking a goal which
recedes as it advances. The individual organism fails
but the race goes on. The immediate goal of the
organism, the most general function of the mind, is
one of attempting the attainment of equilibrium, and
in this word we have again the combination of effort
and failure; for while the mind is constantly reaching
out and exerting all of its forces to balance internal
tensions to relieve the discomfort of stresses, if by
any chance it could succeed it would mean death because the only true equilibrium is a static state of
rest. This energic concept is to my mind one of great
usefulness. I always believed, for example, that
Janet's concept of psychological tension had been too
hastily laid aside, and it seems to me now that it is

all being reëmphasized anew in the Gestalt psychology. Configurations persist in virtue of their inner tensions. The unsolved problem is remembered longer than the solved problem. Phantasy diagrams which are incomplete are dwelt upon until their completion becomes an accomplished fact. Attitudes of mind harass the individual when they contain unsolved problems and continue to do so until the problem reaches some sort of solution and the individual correspondingly some sort of quiescence. These internal stresses and strains constitute what might properly be called stress diagrams that have an inherent tendency of their own to gravitate, as it were, to some state of equilibrium, an expression on the energic side which I suspect is not dissimilar to the psychological expression of anxiety; and I might add to anxiety curiosity as being another of those drives which make for the release of tension. In this connection I think we have as yet missed the opportunity of adequately utilizing the body image as a source of information of internal stresses and an indication of their nature, to inform us further of the mechanisms of intrapsychic activity as they express themselves in these terms. I am happy to see these aspects of psychological problems emphasized in the Gestalt psychology; for I feel that in many ways the different methods of approach to the study of the human mind by the different schools of psychology and the different methodologies have remained too much isolated one from another, although I appreciate that in a sense this degree of segregation of interests is essential in the way of progress. However, the time has come when a tolerant attitude of mind will be open to the reception of the results of research in all these various directions and see in the net results agreements which are of greater significance than the individual accomplishments in each separate instance could possibly be. Whitehead, speaking of Plato, says that: "The moral of his writings is that all points of view, reasonably coherent and in some sense with an application, have something to contribute to our understanding of the universe, and also involve omissions whereby they fail to include the totality of evident fact. The duty of tolerance is our finite homage to the abundance of inexhaustible novelty which is awaiting the future, and to the complexity of accomplished fact which exceeds our strength of insight." My own feeling is that tolerance is the basis upon which that structure of human thinking can be erected that will make for such a mutual appreciation and understanding as will cement human relationships in a way consonant with that further progress in culture that is our main social objective. One who would approach the stupendous problem of the human mind in any other than a tolerant attitude, prepared to give due weight to the opinions of others, is inviting disaster to begin with, which cannot help but result in an enormous amount of lost motion. There has been no time, perhaps, in the history of the world when the opportunities for great accomplishment challenged man's inventive genius more obviously than they do today. There has been no time when traditions, prejudices, biases of all sorts and descriptions, might be so easily swept aside as they can be now; and therefore there is no time like the present for that enlightenment which may come to man by an examination and knowledge of himself to which psychiatry primarily contributes.

In this connection it is well to again call attention to language as the most important medium by way of which not only are valuable traditions and the experiences of the race perpetuated, but biases, prejudices and misconceptions of all manner equally find themselves imbedded in its structure. The function of language is one of the most complex of all human attributes, and while in all probability it originally had little or nothing to do with the conveyance of thought from one person to another but was rather a method of emotional expression, it has acquired its enormous social significance because it has become the most important means of communication. In the course of its development it has grown by laying down processes and developing words which are relatively static forms used for its purposes of expression. These words are not easy to change but their meaning is not so difficult to change, and so in the course of development it is their meanings and not they that have undergone modification. The result is that the forms of language remain relatively fixed while the meanings attached to these forms undergo all manner of modification, and unless one is alert to this process he is very apt to be deceived by the words which are used. Of course it is very important that the word as a symbol should not change with every slight modification of meaning given to it by each individual.[8] The outstanding function of the word as symbol is therefore as an energy carrier, and while it is essential for the coherence and integration of a group that this symbol should remain something to which all can give allegiance, it is this very necessity and this very value which becomes a danger when one either attempts exact expression along scientific lines or undertakes to express something which one feels but which is different from anything with which one has had experience before, but has no new words with which to mold one's thoughts. As Whitehead puts it: "Human life is driven forward by its dim apprehension of notions too general for its existing language." [9] Such words as "life, liberty and the pursuit of happiness" have served for many years as integrating factors in these United States. On the other hand, such words as

[8] White, William A.: *Mechanisms of Character Formation,* New York. The Macmillan Co. 1922.
[9] *Adventures of Ideas.*

"truth," "justice," "beauty," and a host of other abstract terms, while they have had their integrating functions, have been the nuclei for innumerable discussions, different points of view and disputes. To quote Whitehead again: "It is misleading to study the history of ideas without constant remembrance of the struggle of novel thought with the obtuseness of language." [10] It is always important to know what the other individual is really talking about, to get what he is really trying to express rather than merely to understand in a more or less conventional way the words that he utters; and here again there has been a distinct contribution by psychiatry to this understanding, for every patient is being felt more and more to be an individual problem and what he has to say about himself and his difficulties is being realized more and more definitely to be what I have called the language of his disease,[11] which, like any cryptic hieroglyphs, has to be deciphered, translated, and its meaning discovered. It is just in this region of the exquisitely unique and individualistic that psychiatry has, in recent years particularly, by means of the methodology of psychoanalysis, functioned with peculiar significance. And it is just because of the lack of appreciation of these uniquely individual situations that the academic psychology, particularly

[10] *Op. cit.*
[11] White, William A.: *The Meaning of Disease*. Baltimore. Williams & Wilkins Co. 1926. See Chapter X.

of the last century, and the psychometric manifestations of the present, fail to a very considerable extent. Academic psychology pursued its course with the conventional terms of the day, such as "will," "intellect," "emotion," which applied to nobody knew exactly what, and which, each taken out of its setting, was pretty thoroughly dehumanized by the process. It is the same to a considerable extent with the psychometric tendencies which attempt the quantification of abstract qualities, and when this process is done the result is equally dehumanized; for it is difficult to find in tabulations, statistical statements, averages, means and coefficients of correlation much remaining of the human elements that entered into the original problem. And if they are there it is not infrequently due to the personality of the person making the test rather than to the method itself. It would be interesting here to discuss the whole philosophy of measurement about which the mathematicians and the physicists have been so critical regarding us, and which I have mentioned before, but time presses and we are approaching the end of our presentation.[12]

The language which we use should be so constructed as to express the structures and functions with which modern science is dealing. To undertake

[12] See Shuey, Herbert: "Recent Trends in Science and the Development of Modern Typology." *Psychological Review*, Vol. 41, No. 3, May 1934. See page I.

General Implications

to express modern scientific concepts in language formulated at a previous time before these concepts had evolved is an exceedingly precarious procedure, but what is especially unfortunate is that it tends to perpetuate the older and now false notions and therefore to interfere with the understanding of the new. In other words, the medium of expression tends, because of its structure and the traditions which attach to the words, to falsify the concept which it is sought to express. For instance, in talking of the organism-as-a-whole the mere statement of the body-mind problem, which speaks of the body and the mind as equally significant aspects of the organism, uses language which maintains the old distinction between these two aspects in the statement that that distinction no longer exists. As additional examples I might quote the statement that the brain cortex of man is what is responsible for his superiority of attainment and his place in nature. Such a statement would seem to indicate that the cortex might be considered as a separate entity which could be added to or subtracted from the human individual. There is nothing in this language to indicate that the cortex represents the structuralization of the final syntheses and integrations of the total organism, and that the only way in which a cortex can be added to, for example, is as the result of hundreds of thousands and perhaps millions of years of accumulated experience.

We find the same type of error in the literature of the endocrine glands.[18] These glands are spoken of as if they were separate, and one is reminded of the old mosaic theory of the nervous system as composed of reflexes, of the theory of the organism as composed of the sum of its separate organs added together, each one autonomous in its own right. These defects of expression are just as great as the now quite frequently acknowledged defects of the old Faculty psychology. We recognize that there are no faculties. We need to recognize, also, that these other entities as such do not exist, but in the one case as in the other language still carries on the error. I have no doubt that this is a real obstacle in the evolution of our thinking and the expression of our thoughts.[14]

[18] The literature that has grown up about the endocrine glands is especially guilty of these defects. The glands are spoken of as if they were separate and distinct entities which functioned altogether on their own, as it were, and modified one way or another their host, the body. Their discussion does not seem to indicate that while this point of view is, of course, partly true, it is only true in an holistic sense. The endocrines function, and can only function, as parts of the organism. Like the other organs, they represent the nucleated precipitates of certain necessities in the way of function which have become highly specialized and relegated preponderantly to these particular loci.

[14] Korzybski in his recent work, *Science and Sanity*, traces most of the ills from which we suffer to the discrepancy between the structure of language and the structure of

General Implications

I have from time to time in the course of these lectures referred to the desirability of further research. I have mentioned only a certain few directions which this research might profitably take, but I want to emphasize now that the type of research which I personally believe in above all others is research in pure science, not research with some so-called practical goal in sight. Over and over again great scientific truths have been discovered by the genius working to no other end than to enlarge the field of knowledge, and as many times have the results that have flowed from such discoveries not only been unexpected, unpredicted, and unforeseen, but they have been stupendous beyond the most ambitious imagination. Perhaps the only excuse for mentioning this—I think I may say well-known fact as the result of experience in the past—is that so many of our institutions for mental disease, in fact most of them, are supported by public funds, and appropriating bodies are rather apt to feel that their responsibilities compel them to give money where some very concrete and worth while objective is practically within sight.

Finally, there is one further matter which I con-

the universe, as he puts it, and believes that the remedy for these ills lies in correcting this discrepancy.

See also Huse, H. R.: *The Illiteracy of the Literate.* New York. London. D. Appleton-Century Co., Inc. 1933.

sider to be of importance in a field to which again psychiatry has made, I think, a definite contribution. It is still quite the fashion to speak of disease as either functional or organic, and as I have already indicated I do not know how to distinguish these two unless they be distinguished by the characteristics of reversibility or irreversibility; but however that may be, there are certain psychological character-istics which are present as accompaniments of disease processes in either instance, and the fact that the disease is organic need not deter us from undertaking an investigation of these psychological constituents. In fact it may turn out to be of supreme significance to know how organic disease affects psychological reactions. The study of general paresis at the psycho-logical level has been fully justified, even though the disease itself may be considered to be basically organic, irreversible and irrecoverable. We can see under these circumstances, just as we have seen else-where, what I believe to be the outstanding function of the mind, or to put it better, the basically most significant way in which it expresses itself, namely, in the way that all energy expresses itself—and here I am almost forced to use anthropomorphic lan-guage: to seek an equilibrium. The psyche might be considered as an organ for equalizing stresses, re-leasing tensions and thus bringing about, or attempt-ing to bring about, a state of equilibrium.

One of the outstanding illustrations of this effort

at seeking an equilibrium is seen in the paretic delusion of grandeur. This differs from other euphoric attitudes by being expressed in expanding delusions which become so grandiose that there are no existing words to express them. Particularly is this so with reference to the alleged money possessions of the patient. Here the amount of money, which begins by being expressed by millions, soon gets to billions, trillions, sextillions, etc., until the patient loses himself in the effort to set down a large enough figure. This growth of the paretic delusion of grandeur is what I have called the pyramiding of the delusional system and takes place in a futile effort to compensate for the actual physical destruction taking place in the brain. Inasmuch as this compensation can never be attained, the effect continues in this endless fashion to pile up expressions of ever-increasing magnitude.

As you probably have already sensed, my own personal preference for the terminology in the field in which we are moving is the terminology of energy in its various transformations and distributions. Here I think we can take over some of the language of modern physics in our efforts to express our understanding of what is going on in the psyche. For example, I think that the concept of the dynamic gradient as set forth by Child is exceedingly valuable, particularly when we realize that the head end of the organism, in accordance with this theory, is the dominant end, and also that the main function of the head end, namely, the mind, is the most modifiable of all the aspects of the organism, so that we have in the mind not only the most powerful agent at our disposal but the one most readily modified. If our attack upon illness is made by the means of psychotherapy, we may therefore feel that we are not by any means necessarily failing to deal with conditions which have at least heretofore often, if not always, been considered to be organic and therefore irreversible. There are many illustrations within the field of psychotherapy which show that the possibilities of this method are not only not exhausted, but that it may be that we are very far from appreciating their powers. Smuts, the advocate of holism, has said: "So far from biology being forced into a physical mold, the position will in future be reversed. Physics will look to biology and even to psychology for hints, clues and suggestions." [15]

These considerations lead me to speak very briefly of the unconscious in this connection. One of the most important contributions in the whole psychiatric field has been this hypothesis of the unconscious, upon which the technique of psychoanalysis is based. It is essential always to approach any psychiatric problem with this concept of the field of the unconscious systems always in mind. It is never sufficient

[15] Smuts, J. C.: "The Scientific World-Picture of Today." *Science*. September 25, 1931.

to ask a patient if he believes or wishes this or that. His answer confined to the field of clear consciousness is never a sufficient answer, and we have had to learn methods of indirection by which the real answers may be disclosed. With this you are familiar. I have called these systems of the unconscious the "organ of the unconscious," and I feel that perhaps there is a field here for research which is ordinarily not considered because it has implications which make the scientific mind shy away from it. But if our ideas of evolution and development are correct, our ancestors must have looked out upon a very different world from the one which we see. Powers of perception, for example, were probably very much more extensive although in special directions very much less intensive; and as these powers have changed by a contracting of their extensiveness and a deepening of their intensiveness we have lost in proportion to our gains, and quite possibly in certain regressive states powers of perception may be reanimated which produce somewhat startling results. We are familiar, for example, with the increased power of perception of some of the special sense organs when one of the special senses is destroyed. We are also familiar with the phenomena of increased sensual acuity that we used to see from time to time when we were more in the habit of using hypnosis. May I intimate that it is quite possible that what we know of intuition belongs to this twilight zone of somewhat vague perception, that the organ of the unconscious takes in many things which never reach clear consciousness and that the net result which we speak of as intuition may be found to have had its origin in this region? These are some of the implications, psychological in nature, which one draws from the experience of various mentally disordered individuals and which seem to be illuminating.

Then there is the field of language, about which I have already spoken, which gradually comes to incorporate in its forms the experiences of the race for purposes, among others, of communication, and which needs, therefore, to be studied with especial reference to the changing concepts in our field. We are to a very considerable extent, and without knowing it, imprisoned in our ways of thinking by the forms of language; and the fact that this imprisonment is an unconscious one makes it doubly difficult for us to deal with it. For example, in undertaking to deal with the concept of the organism-as-a-whole we insist that the mind-body relationship constitutes a unity, and in the very statement that it is a unity we are bound to use the language which indicates a dualistic point of view. Our language, therefore, thwarts us in progressing along untrodden ways, because we have no means of communicating the things we feel, at least not until we have developed a language which is adequate. I would suggest that as the physicists and the astronomers speak of a time-space manifold so we might express our meaning by hyphenating a number of our terms, such as body-mind, emotion-intellect, heredity-environment, so that the printed word would convey that something more was meant than is ordinarily intended by the use of these words separately.[16]

It will be remembered that years ago Wernicke suggested that aphasia might ultimately become the pattern, the form, which would be used to express the psychoses. It is quite possible that this statement of Wernicke will come true in a way which we least expected at the time it was made and that language, which by its very nature and history is the precipitate not only of our experiences but of our philosophy, which is the medium for the expression of symbols, which symbols are used for purposes of energy transformation, may become increasingly significant and important in our understanding of psychotic reactions. Certainly the study of language, particularly of the various aphasias,[17] is giving us confirmatory evidence of our ideas of the structure of the psyche, is tending to close the gap between the so-called

[16] See Chap. X, "The Language of Disease," in my *Meaning of Disease. Op. cit.*

[17] White, William A.: "The Language of the Psychoses." *The Amer. Jour. of Psychiatry,* Vol. IX, No. 4. January 1930. See also page 165.
Schilder, Paul: "Personality in the Light of Psychoanalysis." *The Psychoanalytic Review,* Vol. XXII, No. 1. January 1935.

"functional" and so-called "organic" and as our new concepts develop further may succeed completely. The parallel lines of the Euclidian geometry, which meet only in infinity, may finally come in the new universe that has grown up within the past generation to meet within finite limitations.

Let me give a simple instance of the value of the energic point of view which I have been discussing. In the agitation for the sterilization of the unfit the constructive possibilities of inadequacies have never been discussed, so far as I know. For example, it never seems to have occurred to anyone engaged in this discussion that some things which are called unfit may have definite and positive values. It has been stated by writers that the neurotic has made valuable contributions to knowledge and to civilization in general. If this is true, then is it not also true that certain undesirable features represented in the germ plasm which lead to neurosis may, if they form part of a particular kind of pattern, not simply produce disastrous results but may produce highly desirable results? For example, certain types of individuals presented with certain internal obstacles develop compensatory reactions which prove of the utmost value to the race. Many of the greatest men who ever lived are credited with having had psychopathic traits. Would one wish to have so thoroughly effected sterilization of the unfit that any constitutional traits which would have led to such results would have been completely destroyed? Is one sufficiently sure that with the destruction of such constitutional traits the marvelous personalities of these great geniuses would have developed as they did? Of course this is purely speculative, but certainly we do know the phenomena of compensation, and we do know that this compensation takes place as the result of inner deficiencies and that it does lead to valuable social results. These are considerations, it seems to me, of the utmost significance.

I have mentioned this tendency particularly in the few words I have said about the stress diagrams as they appeared in the Gestalt psychology. I am mentioning them here again from the general, broad viewpoint of the organism as an energy system which moves forward only so long as it is spurred in that direction by necessity, and which tends, at once that necessity is withdrawn, to lapse into a state of quiescence. The living, functioning organism is an acting organism to which there is continuously presented new problems, difficulties to be overcome. Many of these new problems are presented with a vagueness so great that they can neither be clearly seen nor definitely formulated. They are felt to occupy a region which escapes clear-cut vision and definite formulation, a region which Flower describes as the region of "beyondness." Here is the field in which mysticism holds forth and also, specifically, the field of religion. Let me quote briefly to you from Flower regarding this particular situation: "The environment is perpetually presenting itself in unfamiliar, surprising and perplexing aspects; these features will have, as it were, a halo of 'beyondness' or mystery. But though there is no specific tendency capable of responding to such a situation, involving the discrimination of a complexity beyond the range of predisposition, the urge to make some response is still there, being an intrinsic characteristic of any kind of perceptual experience; and religion is one of the attempts of man to overcome the inadequacy of his innate equipment as he enters into the larger world which is no longer walled round by specific adaptation mechanisms. We may say, then, that the religious response is so far from being the expression of a specific religious tendency or instinct, as some writers have tried to maintain that it is precisely the outcome of the inadequacy of specific response tendencies. It is man's attempt—or one of his attempts—to supplement the paucity of his original endowment when he discovers himself in a strange world." [18]

From this you will see that mankind not only has the problem of meeting reality as we ordinarily know it, dealing with it in an effective way, mastering the environment, as it is called, not only has the dual problems of dealing with the outside world and the world within, but he is in addition faced with what

[18] *The Psychology of Religion.*

the future may hold in store for him, and in his endeavor to encompass this apparently impossible set of circumstances which his own meditations have created he attempts here again to bring to pass certain conditions within his psyche that will make for peace and comfort and which move in the direction of equilibrium.

Whatever may be one's beliefs or convictions in this or any other field, psychiatry has made the valuable contribution of showing something of the mechanisms which are at work in dealing with these various problems, the reasons for their existence and the possibilities for solution which they present, and how those solutions are brought about. The whole field of tradition, of superstition, of bias, the field in which under the disguise of socially accepted terms and activities and conventional language the primitive and destructive instincts of man function and do their will, is here uncovered; and the somewhat commonly accepted situation that civilization itself is threatened because in the past half century or so man has obtained as a result of scientific advance control of his environment with a tremendously accelerating rapidity, whereas his control of himself remains practically at a standstill, is here provided with an actual usable weapon for dealing with this discrepancy, and it is perhaps the most valuable single contribution to the progress of civilization that psychiatric thought has made by its implications in this direction.

In these days of trial through which we have been and still are passing, every thoughtful man from time to time reviews the field, at least that portion of it with which he is best acquainted, and speculates upon the possibilities as he sees them of contributions from this era adding something worth while to the solution of the difficulties as they present themselves. There was a time in the history of this country when all of the possibilities of the future were thought out in terms of western frontier. It was towards the west that man fixed his vision, and there he saw undeveloped resources representing fabulous wealth which lay ready to his hand to develop, and which so far as he could see would supply him in coming generations for a great period of time. The western frontier no longer exists, at least in the sense in which it did in the days of our forefathers; but there is a frontier which exists now as it always has and which because of its obviousness so often escapes recognition. I mean the frontier of the mind, which despite its hundreds of thousands of years of history still presents possibilities that so far as our practical purposes are concerned are infinite. No one has yet dared to suggest a limit to the possibilities of the human mind, and it is to these possibilities that we must turn with an abiding hope and a conviction and assurance that they will not fail us. I will not undertake to elaborate even in general terms what these possibilities are. Any one of you who is at all familiar with the scientific literature will realize as this literature passes before your eyes day by day that the wealth of material with which the mind is dealing in the various departments of science alone is beyond the possibility of any individual mind to grasp. These potentialities are constantly becoming kinetic, and the great field of beyondness as looked at from this point of view contains in fact, as well as in imagination, the satisfaction of all our wishes.

We are surrounded on all sides by the unknown, whether we attempt to penetrate the past or the future or to understand the present. It is the function of science to be everlastingly attempting to push forward its discoveries into these regions of darkness and to illuminate them with knowledge. Even the region of beyondness, which man seems to have set aside for his special purposes to remain sacrosanct to all efforts of this sort, is beginning to yield to scientific pressure. If we look back over the history of the progress of interpreting the universe we will find that man has always relinquished his own right to self-determination, his own particular place in the sun, only with the greatest resistance; and yet it would seem that in this field in which we are interested we have to assume that the principle of determination operates if we are to get anywhere in our efforts. However, you will recall my discussion of this subject and my quotation from Whitehead to the effect that the unrelatedness of contemporary events establishes a region of freedom in the universe, and so perhaps man may be prepared to have all of his activities which in the past have been considered as the free actions of myriads of individuals reduced to law, the operations of natural law such as govern in the other regions of the universe. If he can realize that these laws have their origin in common experience from the depths, the very springs of life, and affect all alike—to be a part of life in its very beginnings, a part of the universe itself in this sense, is by no means to humiliate him, the thought that is implied in the doctrine of determination as ordinarily conceived. We need no longer resent the fact that our motives in their last analysis are of such origin.

There are innumerable matters that might properly receive attention in such a discussion as this, but there are three directions in which I look for progress as a result of psychiatric developments which will lead to important results.

1. In general medicine—the wider and more informed recognition that the relationship between patient and physician constitutes the most important tool of therapy.

2. In general science—the recognition that investigations of the neurological and psychological

foundations of such concepts as space and time constitute an all-important avenue of approach to the elucidation of their deeper meanings and significances.

3. In the field of sociology—the study of the phenomena of and the factors that lie behind war and peace.

In closing this presentation I feel that it is important that the final note should be one that re-emphasizes the tremendous growth of science during the present century, and the extent to which psychiatric thinking has developed and become amalgamated with the advances in thought in all directions which directly or indirectly affect man and his multitudinous activities.

Man has had to repeatedly renounce cherished convictions of his own importance and significance in the universe. His self-regard has been wounded by each dethronement forced upon him by the advances in science. But as compensation for being thus forced to a recognition of his own insignificance he has gradually become, not merely an inhabitant of the universe, organically separate, distinct and apart from its operations except as he may control small bits of it in his immediate neighborhood, but a part of this gigantic affair, infinite in time and space, and a medium through which it is focussed and in accordance with the laws of which he has his being and finds his ways of self-expression. While he has contracted on the one hand he has indefinitely expanded on the other, and instead of just losing his importance he has been reinstated and reënthroned as the central figure in the universe, by and through which the cosmos must, in the last analysis, be interpreted and receive its meanings. By such great pulsations do the tides of human affairs rise and fall.

BIBLIOGRAPHY

THE FOLLOWING IS in no sense an attempt to set forth a bibliography of psychiatry. This would require a volume by itself. I am merely noting herein a sampling of the more important books and articles that have crossed my desk in the past few months, and to which I have had occasion to refer in the preparation of these chapters, in addition to those cited in the footnotes.

Babcock, Harriet, *Dementia Praecox, a Psychological Study*. New York. The Science Press Printing Co. (Lancaster, Pa.) 1933.

Bergson, Henri. *Creative Evolution*. New York. Henry Holt & Co. 1911.

Binet, Alfred, and Simon, Th. *The Intelligence of the Feeble-minded*. Vineland, New Jersey. The Training School. 1916.

———— *The Development of Intelligence in Children* (The Binet-Simon Scale.) Vineland, New Jersey. The Training School. 1916.

Buchanan, S. "Freudian Dynamics." *Psyche*. April 1932.

Campbell, Charles Macfie. *Towards Mental Health, The Schizophrenic Problem*. Cambridge. Harvard University Press. 1933.

Child, C. M. *Individuality in Organisms*. University of Chicago Press. 1915.

———— *Senescence and Rejuvenescence*. University of Chicago Press. 1915.

————"The Basis of Physiological Individuality in Organisms." *Science*. April 14, 1916.

———— *The Origin and Development of the Nervous System from a Physiological Viewpoint*. University of Chicago Press. 1921.

Coghill, G. E. "The Early Development of Behavior in Amblystoma and in Man." *Arch. Neuro. & Psychiatry*. May, 1929.

————"Individuation versus Integration in the Development of Behavior." *Jr. of General Psychology*. 1930.

————"The Structural Basis of the Integration of Behavior." *Proc. National Academy of Sciences*. October 1930.

————"Correlated Anatomical and Physiological

Bibliography

Studies of the Growth of the Nervous System of Amphibia. X. Corollaries of the Anatomical and Physiological Study of Amblystoma from the Age of Earliest Movement to Swimming." *Jr. Comp. Neurol.* August 1931.

———"The Neuro-Embryologic Study of Behavior: Principles, Perspective and Aim." *Science.* August 18, 1933.

———"Growth of a Localized Functional Center in a Relatively Equipotential Nervous Organ." *Arch. Neuro & Psychiatry.* November 1933.

Crichton-Miller, H. *Psycho-Analysis and Its Derivatives.* New York. Henry Holt & Co. 1933.

Denison, J. H. *Emotion as the Basis of Civilization.* New York: London. Charles Scribner's Sons. 1928.

Donnison, C. P. "The Cause of Hyperpiesia. Presentation of a Hypothesis." *British Med. Jr.* April 21, 1934.

Fenichel, Otto. *Outline of Clinical Psychoanalysis.* New York. W. W. Norton & Co. 1934.

Flower, J. Cyril. *An Approach to The Psychology of Religion.* New York. Harcourt, Brace & Co. 1927.

Flugel, J. C. *A Hundred Years of Psychology 1833-1933.* New York. Macmillan Co. 1933.

Gadelius, Bror. *Human Mentality in the Light of Psychiatric Experience. An Outline of General Psychiatry*. London. Humphrey Milford. Oxford University Press. 1933.

Goodenough, Florence L. *Developmental Psychology. An Introduction to the Study of Human Behavior*. New York. D. Appleton-Century Co. 1934.

Heidbreder, Edna. *Seven Psychologies*. New York: London. The Century Co. 1933.

Hinsie, Leland E. *Syllabus of Psychiatry. A Guide to General Orientation*. Utica, N. Y. State Hospitals Press. 1933.

Hull, Clark L. *Hypnosis and Suggestibility. An Experimental Approach*. New York: London. D. Appleton-Century Co. 1933.

Irwin, Orvis C. "The Organismic Hypothesis and Differentiation of Behavior. I. The Cell Theory and the Neurone Doctrine." *Psychological Review*. March 1932.

———"The Organismic Hypothesis and Differentiation of Behavior. II. The Reflex Arc Concept." *Psychological Review*. May 1932.

———"The Organismic Hypothesis and Differentiation of Behavior. III. The Differentiation of Human Behavior." *Psychological Review*. July 1932.

Bibliography

Jennings, H. S. *Prometheus, or Biology and the Advancement of Man.* New York. E. P. Dutton & Co. 1925.

Josey, Charles Conant. *The Social Philosophy of Instinct.* New York. Charles Scribner's Sons. 1922.

Köhler, Wolfgang. *Gestalt Psychology.* New York. Horace Liveright. 1929.

Kretschmer, E. *Physique and Character. An Investigation of the Nature of Constitution and of the Theory of Temperament.* New York, Harcourt, Brace & Co. 1925.

Lowie, Robert H. *Primitive Society.* New York. Boni & Liveright. 1920.

Luria, A. R. *The Nature of Human Conflicts, or Emotion, Conflict and Will. An Objective Study or Disorganization and Control of Human Behavior.* New York. Liveright. 1932.

Nicole, J. Ernest. *Psychopathology, a Survey of Modern Approaches.* Baltimore. William Wood & Co. 1934.

Ogburn, William Fielding. *Social Change with Respect to Culture and Original Nature.* New York. B. W. Huebsch. 1922.

Penrose, Lionel S. *Mental Defect.* New York. Farrar & Rinehart. 1934.

Rothschild, Richard. *Reality and Illusion. A New Framework of Values.* New York. Harcourt, Brace & Co. 1934.

Salmon, Thomas W. "The Insane in a County Poor Farm." *Mental Hygiene,* Vol. 1, p. 25. January 1917.
————*Mind and Medicine.* New York. Columbia University Press. 1924.

Schiller, F.C.S. *Riddles of the Sphinx. A Study in the Philosophy of Humanism.* London. Macmillan Co. 1912.

Schwesinger, Gladys C. *Heredity and Environment. Studies in the Genesis of Psychological Characteristics.* New York. Macmillan Co. 1933.

Smuts, J. C. "The Scientific World-Picture of To-Day." *Science,* Sept. 25, 1931.

Spengler, Oswald. "The Downfall of Western Civilization." *The Dial,* November 1924; December 1924; January 1925.

Stevenson, George S., and Smith, Geddes. *Child Guidance Clinics, A Quarter Century of Development.* New York. The Commonwealth Fund. 1934.

Stockard, Charles R. *The Physical Basis of Personality.* New York. W. W. Norton & Co. 1931.

Vaihinger, H. *The Philosophy of "As If." A System of the Theoretical, Practical and Religious Fic-*

tions of Mankind. New York. Harcourt, Brace & Co. 1925.

Wheeler, Raymond Holder, and Perkins, Francis Theodore. *Principles of Mental Development. A Textbook in Educational Psychology*. New York. Thomas Y. Crowell Co. 1932.

White, William A. *Insanity and the Criminal Law*. New York. Macmillan. 1923.

———— *The Meaning of Disease. An Inquiry in the Field of Medical Philosophy*. Baltimore. Williams & Wilkins Co. 1926.

———— *Medical Psychology. The Mental Factor in Disease*. Washington. Nervous and Mental Disease Pub. Co. 1931.

———— *Forty Years of Psychiatry*. Washington. Nervous and Mental Disease Pub. Co. 1933.

———— *Crimes and Criminals*. New York. Farrar & Rinehart. 1933.

Whitehead, A. N. *An Introduction to Mathematics*. New York. Henry Holt & Co. 1911.

———— *Adventures of Ideas*. New York. Macmillan Co. 1933.

Witty, Paul A., and Lehman, Harvey C. "The Instinct Hypothesis *versus* the Maturation Hypothesis." *Psychological Review*. January 1933.

INDEX

Index

Index

Index

Index

Index

MENTAL ILLNESS AND SOCIAL POLICY
The American Experience

An Arno Press Collection

Barr, Martin W. Mental Defectives: Their History, Treatment and Training. 1904.

The Beginnings of American Psychiatric Thought and Practice: Five Accounts, 1811-1830. 1973

The Beginnings of Mental Hygiene in America: Three Selected Essays, 1833-1850. 1973

Briggs, L. Vernon, et al. History of the Psychopathic Hospital, Boston, Massachusetts. 1922

Briggs, L. Vernon. Occupation as a Substitute for Restraint in the Treatment of the Mentally Ill. 1923

Brigham, Amariah. An Inquiry Concerning the Diseases and Functions of the Brain, the Spinal Cord, and the Nerves. 1840

Brigham, Amariah. Observations on the Influence of Religion upon the Health and Physical Welfare of Mankind. 1835

Brill, A. A. Fundamental Conceptions of Psychoanalysis. 1921

Bucknill, John Charles. Notes on Asylums for the Insane in America. 1876

Conolly, John. The Treatment of the Insane Without Mechanical Restraints. 1856

Coriat, Isador H. What is Psychoanalysis? 1917

Deutsch, Albert. The Shame of the States. 1948

Dewey, Richard. Recollections of Richard Dewey: Pioneer in American Psychiatry. 1936

Earle, Pliny. Memoirs of Pliny Earle, M. D. with Extracts from his Diary and Letters (1830-1892) and Selections from his Professional Writings (1839-1891). 1898

Galt, John M. The Treatment of Insanity. 1846

Goddard, Henry Herbert. Feeble-mindedness: Its Causes and Consequences. 1926

Hammond, William A. A Treatise on Insanity in Its Medical Relations. 1883

Hazard, Thomas R. Report on the Poor and Insane in Rhode-Island. 1851

Hurd, Henry M., editor. The Institutional Care of the Insane in the United States and Canada. 1916/1917. Four volumes.

Kirkbride, Thomas S. On the Construction, Organization, and General Arrangements of Hospitals for the Insane. 1880

Meyer, Adolf. The Commonsense Psychiatry of Dr. Adolf Meyer: Fifty-two Selected Papers. 1948

Mitchell, S. Weir. Wear and Tear, or Hints for the Overworked. 1887

Morton, Thomas G. The History of the Pennsylvania Hospital, 1751-1895. 1895

Ordronaux, John. Jurisprudence in Medicine in Relation to the Law. 1869

The Origins of the State Mental Hospital in America: Six Documentary Studies, 1837-1856. 1973

Packard, Mrs. E. P. W. Modern Persecution, or Insane Asylums Unveiled, As Demonstrated by the Report of the Investigating Committee of the Legislature of Illinois. 1875. Two volumes in one

Prichard, James C. A Treatise on Insanity and Other Disorders Affecting the Mind. 1837

Prince, Morton. The Unconscious: The Fundamentals of Human Personality Normal and Abnormal. 1921

Putnam, James Jackson. Human Motives. 1915

Russell, William Logie. The New York Hospital: A History of the Psychiatric Service, 1771-1936. 1945

Sidis, Boris. The Psychology of Suggestion: A Research into the Subconscious Nature of Man and Society. 1899

Southard, Elmer E. Shell-Shock and Other Neuropsychiatric Problems Presented in Five Hundred and Eighty-Nine Case Histories from the War Literature, 1914-1918. 1919

Southard, E[lmer] E. and Mary C. Jarrett. The Kingdom of Evils. 1922

Southard, E[lmer] E. and H[arry] C. Solomon. Neurosyphilis: Modern Systematic Diagnosis and Treatment Presented in One Hundred and Thirty-seven Case Histories. 1917

Spitzka, E[dward] C. Insanity: Its Classification, Diagnosis and Treatment. 1887

Supreme Court Holding a Criminal Term, No. 14056. The United States vs. Charles J. Guiteau. 1881/1882. Two volumes

Trezevant, Daniel H. Letters to his Excellency Governor Manning on the Lunatic Asylum. 1854

Tuke, D[aniel] Hack. The Insane in the United States and Canada. 1885

Upham, Thomas C. Outlines of Imperfect and Disordered Mental Action. 1868

White, William A[lanson]. Twentieth Century Psychiatry: Its Contribution to Man's Knowledge of Himself. 1936

Willard, Sylvester D. Report on the Condition of the Insane Poor in the County Poor Houses of New York. 1865